10/99

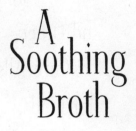

A Soothing Broth

Tonics,

Custards,

Soups,

and Other

Cure-Alls

for Colds,

Coughs,

Upset Tummies,

and

Out-of-Sorts

Days

A Soothing Broth

Pat Willard

BROADWAY BOOKS   NEW YORK

This book contains general reference information about folk cures, remedies, and feeding the ill. It is not intended as a substitute for the advice and care of a physician, and the reader should use proper discretion in utilizing the information and recipes presented. The publisher and the author disclaim liability arising directly or indirectly from the use of the book.

A SOOTHING BROTH. Copyright © 1998 by Pat Willard. All rights reserved. Printed in the United States of America. No part of this book may be reproduced or transmitted in any form or by any means, electronic or mechanical, including photocopying, recording, or by any information storage and retrieval system, without written permission from the publisher. For information, address Broadway Books, a division of Bantam Doubleday Dell Publishing Group, Inc., 1540 Broadway, New York, NY 10036.

Broadway Books titles may be purchased for business or promotional use or for special sales. For information, please write to: Special Markets Department, Bantam Doubleday Dell Publishing Group, Inc., 1540 Broadway, New York, NY 10036.

BROADWAY BOOKS and its logo, a letter B bisected on the diagonal, are trademarks of Broadway Books, a division of Bantam Doubleday Dell Publishing Group, Inc.

Designed by Mauna Eichner

Library of Congress Cataloging-in-Publication Data

Willard, Pat.
A soothing broth : tonics, custards, soups, and other cure-alls for colds, coughs, upset tummies, and out-of-sorts days / Pat Willard. — 1st ed.
p.   cm.
Includes bibliographical references and index.
ISBN 0-7679-0148-7 (hardcover)
1. Liquid diet.   2. Soups—Therapeutic use.   3. Tonics (Medicinal preparations)
I. Title.
RM239.W54   1999
615.8'54—DC21   98-9281
CIP

FIRST EDITION

98 99 00 01 02 10 9 8 7 6 5 4 3 2 1

For my sister,
Suzanne

Acknowledgments

I would foremost like to thank Sue Willard Gregonis, Assistant Professor of Nursing, Allegheny University, for her thorough clinical reading and editing of the manuscript and recipes, for introducing me to Florence Nightingale, and for her humor, guidance, and insight into nursing lore. Thanks to the Visiting Nurse Society of Philadelphia Records, Center for the Study of the History of Nursing, School of Nursing, University of Pennsylvania, for permission to use their archives. Finally, I would like to express my deep appreciation to my editor, Harriet Bell, for seeing the worth, and taking a chance, with these forgotten gems.

Permissions

Grateful acknowledgment is made to the following to reprint their recipes:

"Banana Flip" and "Sulphur and Treacle" from *The Scottish Bakehouse Cook Book* by Isabella M. White, Tashmoo Press, Martha's Vineyard, MA.

"Saffron Consommé" from *The Pleasures of Cooking* magazine. Carl G. Sontheimer, Cuisinart Cooking Club, Inc.

Contents

The Klutz
Beside the Bed

I was twenty-three years old and not long married when my husband became seriously ill. We had moved to New York a few months earlier, into a small apartment overlooking a narrow air shaft, near the university where Chris was to study for his master's degree. While he went to classes and the library, I tramped around looking for a job. Just in the first two months I was a secretary for a stockbroker, a receptionist at a trade organization, and a seamstress for a very expensive interior designer. Each job paid a little better than the last, but we were still living on next to nothing.

When I left for work early one rainy October morning, Chris was still in bed. He had been up late studying the night before and I recalled that, when he tumbled in beside me, he complained of a headache. As I got ready to leave, he mumbled to me to bring home something for his throat; it was scratchy. He told me he had another hour before his class met and I kissed him goodbye.

Nine hours later, I returned to find him still in bed. Or rather, across the bed, the sheets twisted around him and the mattress soaked under his body. The green T-shirt he wore seemed black with sweat. As I walked toward him, Chris started screaming about the bugs that were all around the room. They were crawling up the wall, on the ceiling, trailing light behind them. I crouched down beside the bed and felt the heat rising off his skin. I knew he hadn't made it to class. A fastidious man, he was unshaven, unwashed, and his eyeglasses were nowhere to be found.

I touched his forehead, then jumped away. I don't think I have ever felt anything as hot before, certainly nothing that was alive. I ran into the bathroom, searching for a thermometer. When I returned to take his temperature, he was violently pushing the covers away.

"They're hurting me," he complained, his tone both irritated and desperate for relief.

I got him to lie down and hold the thermometer in his mouth. As I waited, I stroked his face and he relaxed—almost collapsed, really. The thermometer read 105°F. I immediately made him swallow some aspirin and drink a large glass of orange juice. Ten minutes later, Chris threw up the juice. I forced one more aspirin into him—this time with water. Then he passed out.

I changed the top sheet on the bed, put a cold washcloth on his forehead, then sat by his side, wondering what to do next. I counted out the small amount of money we had on hand. The school's clinic was closed for the night. I didn't know a doctor; we had no health insurance and the thought of dragging Chris the four blocks to the nearest emergency room at what was now close to midnight seemed too daunting. Every four hours I shook Chris awake to give him more aspirin. He barely recognized me. The night stretched on, one of the loneliest I've ever passed, with only growing panic to keep me company. I forgot about all the arguments we ever had or the few small doubts I occasionally harbored about our union, and just yearned for some assurance that Chris would still be with me in the morning.

I tried to pass the hours of my watch by grazing through the stack of nineteenth-century novels I was reading at the time, books in which illness and death were as much a part of family life as any other household event. What I wanted was the decisive knowledge these people had to take care of those who needed them. I wished for Marmee's poise as she tended her daughters in *Little Women,* and I longed for the confidence of Lydgate administering to his patients before his fall from grace in *Middlemarch.* In contrast, I felt myself standing on a distant shore, watching my husband struggle under the waves of his fever. I felt there was nothing I could do that would bring him back safely to me.

By early morning, his fever fell to 101°F. I sponged his body down with warm water, changed the sheets again, and helped him into a clean shirt. Then, after I called work to say I wouldn't be coming in, I climbed into bed beside him and we both fell into a deep sleep that lasted the whole day.

What Chris experienced turned out to be little more than a particularly virulent flu. His fever never got so high again, but he was weak and miserable for a few weeks afterward. I cared for him the way I remembered my own mother caring for our family. I took Chris bowls of Campbell's chicken noodle soup with saltine crackers and glasses of flat ginger ale. At night I brewed him what my mom called "Gallagher's Nyquil"—a cup of weak tea with two tablespoons of honey and a vast quantity of whiskey stirred into it.

This was the best I could do for him, and he survived, but the memory of that night continued to haunt me. We were lucky in that we were two very healthy young animals; neither of us has ever gotten that sick again. But I remained convinced that there was something more I could have done for Chris, and I was determined to find out. In my continuing reading through old novels I caught tantalizing bits of information—teas made of beef, broths fortified with wine, and steaming milk custards with bits of toast floating on top. Surely, I thought, these were preferable to canned soup. But that was all I could find about them, names in books, administered by wise and calm women in crinolines who moved with assurance around the intricacies of the sickroom.

IT TOOK SEVERAL more years of burrowing through books in libraries and second-hand bookstores, church bazaars, and stoop sales to find what I was looking for. Up until the early years of the twentieth century, when medical care was removed from the home and firmly established within hospital walls, there was a branch of food preparation known as invalid cooking. Almost every household cookbook had a section devoted to dishes that were expressly for the sick, all accompanied by helpful hints on when to administer them. Not all the recipes were enticing. Until I tasted it, I couldn't see how Irish moss (a seaweed that when added to broths and custards imparts a gelatinous effect) could be tasted with anything but revulsion. Others, especially those based on vast quantities of wine and liquor (as much as I love the stuff) seemed to me to be of dubious worth. And yet, as I gathered these recipes and tried them out—first on Chris, who was a happy guinea pig whenever he caught the slightest bug, and then my children, who have been afflicted with almost every childhood infirmity known to day-care workers—I began to distinguish the mending strength and real comfort that some of these recipes provided.

About this time, I was also introduced to Florence Nightingale's *Notes on Nursing*. First published in 1860, the book was written to dispense "hints for thought to women who have personal charge of the health of others . . . knowledge which everyone ought to have." A catalog of sound, no-nonsense advice, the book outlines practical instructions, covering everything from the arrangement of household furnishings to the emotional and intellectual requirements needed to tend the sick. Florence Nightingale comes through these pages as a strong force of nature, not at all the demure lady with the lamp I remember being told about as a young girl. In truth, I fell in love with this more challenging, complex woman. Her writing is viciously witty and intelligent, and yet centered on so much common sense and wisdom that I began to feel confident about caring for my family with her advice. (Most of her writings, especially *Notes on Nursing*, remain required reading for nursing students today.)

Although Nightingale did not record any recipes, she held strong opinions about food. Feeding the sick, she claimed, was about seduction. Suffering from a delicate stomach that may be accompanied by nausea, patients often reject food, but it nevertheless must be consumed for the body to regain its strength. "Every careful observer of the sick will agree in this that thousands of patients are annually starved in the midst of plenty, from want of attention to the ways which alone make it possible for them to take food," she said, making me think of the horrible little pale puddles and brownish lumps of matter that regularly arrive on hospital meal trays. It is imperative, Nightingale asserted, that the patient's appetite be courted and that each meal be offered as if it were "a young lady being presented at a ball." As the beautiful daughter of a wealthy family, who had been unwillingly carted from one ball to the next in her parents' vain hope that she'd settle down with a suitable husband and forget her wayward aspirations, Nightingale chose a rather poignant, yet very apt, image. The central quandary of caring for the sick is that, despite the queasy state of their stomachs, they must be fed. To this end, they should be offered dishes that entice the appetite, if not thoroughly relieve the symptoms, and will not hinder their recovery. The ingredients should be the best and the freshest available, the dishes prepared with utmost skill. "Remember that sick cookery should do half the work of your poor patient's weak digestion," she warned. Beyond the actual flavor of the food, equal thought should be given to how it appears and how it is served. Nightingale recommended that meals be served punctually at regular intervals, in small quantities, and presented on a pretty tray set with the best china. (Mary Boland Pequignot, the head of nursing at Johns Hopkins University in 1893, concurred. In her book, *A Handbook of Invalid Cooking*, she declares that, "The invalid tray should be a dainty Dresden watercolor of delicate hues and harmonious tints.") When the patient was through eating, the tray was to be removed from the room quickly to prevent the lingering scent of food from upsetting the patient's stomach. If little or nothing on the tray was touched, another attempt should be made in an hour with another dish, perhaps something as flagrantly flirtatious as a sweet custard or flavored crushed ice.

With the onset of an illness, Miss Nightingale's advice on giving the patient teas and clear broths or consommé remains appropriate. Teas can vary from a weak black brew with milk and lots of sugar, which will revive flagging spirits, or green Chinese teas to calm jumpy nerves, to chamomile to reduce stress or upset-stomach-settling sassafras. Clear broths, beef teas (essentially a weak bouillon made from good-quality flank steak), or consommé maintain the patient's nutritional needs and replenish lost fluids. If there's a fever or the throat is raw, these liquids can be frozen and chopped into a sort of slush to sip through a straw or from a spoon.

Fresh lemon, grapefruit, or orange juices diluted with water or seltzer and served in a tall glass over plenty of cracked ice are most welcome in the afternoon. For dinner, start with toast, dry for the part of the illness when the patient is most nauseous, or maybe dusted with cinnamon sugar or lightly spread with honey. As the illness subsides, and fever or congestion lessen, the menu should concentrate on dishes which will help to rebuild the patient's strength: oatmeal gruels sweetened with brown sugar and honey; shirred eggs; pasta with finely chopped vegetables and cream or cheese stirred in; delicately poached chicken or white fish dampened with a little wine sauce. Before the patient goes off to sleep, a toddy of hot liquid is often beneficial—anything from herbal tea to warm milk flavored with a teaspoon of wine or brandy.

THE SUCCESS I HAD with these recipes and the intense joy I felt in finding a way to nourish my family, made me wonder why invalid cooking—and general home nursing knowledge as a whole—was so thoroughly mislaid. Part of the answer, of course, was the growing acceptance of hospitals. After the Crimean War, advancements in medical procedures, along with improvements in sanitation and building design, transformed hospitals from institutions of last resort to facilities promoting the best care for even the most routine complaints. In the mid 1800s, the medical professions were organized into societies with the express purpose of standardizing and enhancing medical training, as well as improving the general health of the population. In order to survive economically, the (all-male) members of these societies (among them the American Medical Association, founded in 1846) deemed it important that reliance on lay care-givers who were primarily women—wives and mothers, dutiful daughters, unmarried sisters, female religious orders, reformed prostitutes, and working-class girls without families—be discouraged. Professional doctors were helped by the very real advances in medicine that occurred in the first half of this century, particularly with the development of potent antibiotics, against which old family recipes and nursing habits appeared quaint, if not downright foolish. It was rare indeed to find anyone steeping a cup of beef tea after World War II. Fewer diseases ravaged technologically advanced countries; infant mortality declined. The intimate face of serious illness and death became foreign, in a sense even a little shameful, an aberration in our modern world.

Growing up in the 1960s, I rarely came into contact with anything beyond the usual bouts of childhood disorders and winter colds. In fact, illness was not acknowledged at all in my house. My mother was a firm believer in penicillin and the latest fad on the drugstore shelf. When my brother and sister and I came down with something, we were given pills, along with canned chicken soup, and expected to go on as if nothing was the matter. I entered adulthood, married, and began to have children without any knowledge of how to take care of anyone. It is the same with most people today. One of the parents at my son's nursery school once told me that she didn't feel quite prepared for winter until her doctor gave her a prescription for a huge bottle of amoxicillin (universally known in day-care circles as "bubble-gum medicine" for its candy pink color and sweet flavor). Her daughter was prone to ear infections, and at the slightest sniffle the mother began spooning the stuff into her, so afraid, she said, that the illness would progress and her daughter would suffer. Hearing this, I thought of something I had read from a wise doctor who equated the prevalent reliance on antibiotics with the use of napalm during the Vietnam War. Both will certainly wipe out the target but, along the way, much that is good will be destroyed as well.

As I researched further into invalid cooking and listened to the stories other people told me of their own bumbling efforts to nurse their loved ones, I began to understand what had truly been lost. The ritual of invalid cooking, and the practice of caring that Florence Nightingale and others like her advised, seemed to pave the way to a more sensible method of attending to my family's health. But I am the first to admit how often it conflicts with the reality of modern life. In Nightingale's time it was assumed that someone remained at home to prepare and serve these dishes. These days, that's not always true. For many years, especially when my children were small, both my husband and I worked full-time, away from home—a state of affairs that, in this country, is not conducive to caring for the sick. During one particularly memorable winter, there was always at least one person in our family who was desperately ill at home. Our bosses, fairly compassionate men, tolerated a little of the mayhem, but for the most part it was a private struggle to administer the kind of care needed. When neither Chris nor I could take the time off to attend whichever child or spouse was sick, we juggled appointments, thought up lame excuses to leave early, and shamelessly coerced friends and family to pitch in.

Somehow we managed, but it was, and continues to be, an effort, magnified these days by the varying natures of managed care groups, shortened hospital stays, and the danger of insufficient health insurance. The swift, scary illnesses that once ravaged my babies have been replaced by my parents' growing frailties, as well as the increasing realization of my own aging. And yet I rarely experience the kind of panic I felt while I watched over Chris that night. The simple lessons I have learned from the pages of old and weathered cookbooks have taught me much about heeding the necessary conditions of life and the humble wisdom that resides in the balm of a soothing broth.

A Teaspoon of Gum Arabic, a Pinch of Albumen

Tracking Down References and Sources for Invalid Cooking

At first glance, much of invalid cooking may seem baffling. Not a few of the ingredients are strange (perhaps even revolting), the medical practices somewhat questionable, and many of the personalities rightly labeled eccentric.

And yet it would be wrong to dismiss these recipes as obsolete. Examined under modern lights, in the face of our rapidly transforming (some would say deteriorating) health care system, much of invalid cooking holds up to strong scrutiny. Certainly, none of these dishes are meant to supplant prescribed medicine, but prepared carefully and used judicially, most of invalid cooking proves to be a valuable healing ally, particularly beneficial in the management of symptoms.

Modern wisdom does, however, dictate caution. The use of un-cooked egg whites is especially questionable. It's the opinion of the National Egg Board that salmonella poisoning from eating uncooked eggs was responsible for many deaths before its dangers were known. Its victims, particularly infants, the elderly, and anyone with compro-mised immune systems were often the principal recipients of invalid cooking. But eggs are one of the most perfect foods, high in all the es-sential vitamins (except C), as well as most of the essential minerals, especially iron. They are, also, depending on how they are prepared, easy to digest. Instead of throwing out all of the recipes that use raw eggs (which would be a considerable number) the egg board recom-mends cooking yolks and whites until they reach 160°F to ensure that salmonella bacteria have been killed, and I have used this technique in this book. If you don't own one, go out and purchase a good, in-stant-read food thermometer. Even when they are intended for drinks (such as eggnogs or flips—basically fortified shakes), cooking the egg slightly does not noticeably alter the taste. It's another step to add, but the results guarantee safer food for your loved ones.

Yolks: In a heavy saucepan, stir the egg yolk with the liquid from the recipe, at least 2 tablespoons liquid per yolk. (If the recipe does not have any other liquid, use water.) Cook over very low heat, stirring constantly, until the mixture coats a spoon with a thin film, or the temperature on an instant-read thermometer reaches 160°F. The mixture will resemble a thin custard. Cool quickly, either by placing the saucepan directly in a large bowl filled with ice water or putting it in the freezer for a few minutes.

Whites: Place the egg whites in a heavy saucepan or double boiler with the sugar, if any, from the recipe, along with 1 teaspoon water per egg white. If the recipe calls for beating the whites to stiff peaks, add ⅛ teaspoon cream of tartar for every 2 whites. Whisk together and cook over very low heat until the whites reach 160°F. Pour into a large bowl. The whites can now either be beaten to stiff peaks or used directly in the recipe.

It's also important to cook all raw meat thoroughly to kill any *e. coli* bacteria lurking about. Many of the original recipes and guides said that bloody raw beef was a good source of vitamins. (In my research, not a few doctors—but, interestingly enough, none of the nurses and women writers—recommended drinking animal blood for strengthening weak constitutions.) I have changed every direction for raw meat to make sure it is thoroughly cooked. While the initial preparations for beef tea call for the meat to be raw, the resulting liquid is always heated to the boiling point.

The prevalent use of spirits and wines may also be of concern to some readers. With a strong history of alcoholism in my family, I'm very mindful of what alcohol can do, and yet it does promote some beneficial effects, primarily lifting the spirits and bringing a sense of warmth and comfort to the afflicted. The small amounts called for in these recipes are mostly harmless, yet I would continue to advise the readers to use their discretion. Be judicious and prudent, noting that what would be considered a trace amount of liquor to a healthy person is often a wallop to someone with a weakened constitution. If the patient is a recovering alcoholic, omit all alcohol. Giving children beverages or food with alcohol is another real concern. I've used a few of these recipes, particularly the cough remedies and the wine jellies for upset stomachs, on my own children, but not often and certainly not for long periods of time. Usually, I give these preparations at night or late in the afternoon—one or two doses, totaling 2 teaspoons of sweet liquor or wine. That's it. The results were that my children were made more comfortable, and neither of them seems to crave spirits any more than their heritage might predict.

For other recipes, I have given the modern counterparts to ingredients that are either no longer in general use or for which there are now more convenient forms available. Some of these recipes—and they are clearly noted—are not meant to be used. Instead, I have recorded them here merely for their historical interest, without any attempt at a modern translation.

That said, I have found most other recipes with strange ingredients to be beneficial and even delicious. With a little searching, especially in out-of-the-way places (such as in a good herb, health food, or co-op store), you'll be able to find everything you need. Below is a list describing some of the more unusual items, along with further suggestions on where to find them.

Agrimony: An herb also called church steeples, cocklebur, or sticklewort. It is widely available in France as a tea, often drunk as a mealtime beverage. It has a very long and distinguished medical history, dating back to Roman times, and is particularly good for liver complaints due to overeating and drinking.

Albumen: Old-fashioned word for egg whites. Whenever egg whites are added to something, it is said to be albumenized or given an additional boost of protein.

Arrowroot: The starchy product of the arrowroot tuber. It is prized as being a relatively tasteless thickening agent. For invalids, it is very easily digested and helps relieve constipation.

Benzoate lard: Lard mixed with salt of benzoic acid. Used most frequently as a base for liniment. Available in some health food catalogs.

Gum arabic: A product of the bark of certain varieties of acacia trees. Colorless, tasteless, and odorless, it's used as a thickening agent. Can be obtained from specialty bakery shops and catalogs.

Hartshorn: Ammonium bicarbonate, a precursor of baking powder and baking soda. Sold in solid blocks in drugstores, it is ground to powder for use in cooking.

Irish moss: Also known as carrageen, this seaweed is found on both the west coast of Ireland and the Atlantic coast of America. Rich source of iodine. Used as a thickening agent. Found in specialty stores and catalogs.

Pearl barley: Barley with the bran removed. The granulars are steamed and polished. It comes in three sizes—coarse, medium, and fine. Use the fine size in these recipes. Can be found in large supermarkets and good specialty stores.

Rennet: Modern term is junket. It is a coagulating enzyme obtained from the fourth stomach of a young calf. Used to curdle milk for cheeses and to make custards and puddings. It is generally available as a tablet or in a powdered form in large supermarkets and specialty stores.

Resin: Generally meant to be the resin from pine trees (known as rosin). Used as a lubricant. Although it is hard to find, some natural food and health stores carry it.

Rose water: (also orange flower water): A distillation of flower petals that has an intense perfumey flavor and fragrance. Available in health food and some ethnic grocery stores (Indian and Mexican stores, in particular).

Mail Order Sources

Whether buying food, herbs, spices, or other ingredients, purchase the freshest ones possible. If they are packaged, look to see if there is an expiration date. Some herbs come in different forms—pills, capsules, oils, liquids, and crushed leaves. Teas can be made from any of these (including the oil, but it will be, well, oily). Make sure you buy the precise herb you're looking for. Many have similar names and might very well produce the opposite effect to the one you're looking for.

HERBS

Penzeys, Ltd., P.O. Box 933, Muskego, WI 53150. Telephone: 414-679-7207. Fax: 414-679-7878. Quality spices and herbs. Catalog available.

Avena Botanicals, 219 Mill Street, Rockport, ME 04856. Telephone: 207-594-0694. Fax: 207-594-2975. Organically grown and wild-harvested medicinal herbs.

Pacific Botanicals, 4350 Fish Hatchery Road, Grants Pass, OR 97527. Telephone: 541-479-7777. Fax: 541-479-5271. Catalog available.

Boiron-Borneman, 6 Campus Blvd., Building A, Newtown Square, PA 19073. Telephone: (800)-BLU-TUBE. Fax: 800-999-4373. One of the better suppliers of homeopathic remedies.

FLOWER ESSENCES

Flower Essence Services, P.O. Box 1769, Nevada City, CA 95959. Telephone: 530-265-0258. Fax: 530-265-6467. The best source for hundreds of flower essences.

BAKING SUPPLIES

King Arthur Flour Baker's Catalog, P.O. Box 876, Norwich, VT 05055-0876. Telephone: 800-777-4434. One of the best sources for different types of flours, grains, and yeasts.

Dean and DeLuca, 560 Broadway, New York, NY 10012. Telephone: 212-226-6800. Offers flours, hard-to-find baking ingredients, and equipment.

The Vermont Country Store, P.O. Box 3000, Manchester Ctr., VT 05255-3000. Telephone: 802-362-2400. Baking ingredients, health liniments, and potions.

Food History Products, P.O. Box 366, Cherry Hill, NY 13320. Telephone: 607-264-8056. Fax: 607-264-8056. A terrific source for historic food products from the publication, *Food History News*, itself a fascinating newsletter for anyone interested in old recipes. For subscription information, write *Food History News*, S. L. Oliver, editor, HCR 60 Box 354A, Islesboro, ME 04848.

A Trembling in the Head

Headaches, Dizziness,
Fainting, Fevers

When it comes to feeling ill, most people I know fall into one of two behavioral categories, which I think of in military terms: They are either soldiers or deserters. In response to experience and wisdom, some people switch from one to the other, depending on their age and circumstances, but in general our nature dictates the kind of patient we become. Soldiers are the ones who march onward, simply doing what they have to do, ignoring every sign that something is not right. Deserters, on the other hand, skip out at the first rumble. And while it's been my experience that the sexes divide equally among these two categories at any given time, it's often been popular (especially in invalid cooking literature) to think exclusively of men as soldiers and women as deserters.

You would have a hard time convincing me that the first person to voice this opinion was not a man—and probably a doctor, to boot. Early medical textbooks have often portrayed the female as owning a delicate constitution, one that would falter at the least disturbance. Most of these illnesses fell under the diagnoses of "female complaints," which seemed to have encompassed everything from menstrual distress to boredom. The biggest category in this broad area was "nerve"-related, the so-called nervous state manifesting itself in headaches, fainting spells, and a general, although mysterious, weakness of the body. The literature of the last century is filled with examples of women whittling away at life in service to odd and frequently doubted debilities. In discussing the figure of Eva's invalid mother, Marie, in *Uncle Tom's Cabin*, Harriet Beecher Stowe expressed the popular notion that women "suffer . . . the sins of the beloved in their own bodies," a spiritual concept that dovetailed very nicely into popular medical theories about the weaker sex. Women both fought and sanctioned this view, often using their expected weaknesses as a way to opt out of oppressive situations, everything from unhappy marriages and strict social codes to unfulfilled ambitions. Doctors didn't help a bit when the most common course of action was to prescribe a bracing dose of powerful narcotics—cocaine, opium, and laudanum being among the most favored—to which women frequently became addicted.

The women who succumbed to this situation were not always the naive or weak-willed simps that we with our modern sensibilities supposed them to be. Florence Nightingale, whose response to a difficult living situation was to take to her bed with what her doctors called "neurasthenic malfunction," was a prime example of this misconception. The beautiful youngest daughter of extremely wealthy titled landowners, Florence was expected to follow her mother's course in life, namely to marry well and establish a successful social life. After the age of sixteen, the most taxing intellectual accomplishment she could look forward to achieving was the planning and execution of a week in the country for an array of prominent friends.

There was no reason to assume she would wish to do otherwise. Aside from her looks, she knew how to dress, danced very well, and more than held up her end of a dinner conversation. That she was far more intelligent than most people around her was viewed as a slight inconvenience. Her mother claimed it was something they would have to overlook—not that she wanted Florence to act stupid but, as she told a relative, her daughter would simply have to learn *not* to discuss so much. And, for awhile, Florence tried. She shopped in Paris, dutifully made the rounds of country homes, and spent the London season going to concerts and balls. By the time she was twenty-five, she had received several proposals and thought very seriously of marrying one of her suitors, but she longed to do something more. She responded to a voice in her head, which she ascribed to God, who told her it was her duty to devote her life to caring for the sick. If she heard of a stricken servant or relative, she would drop whatever engagements she had (much to the bewilderment of her hostess and family) and tend to the patient in the sick room, unbearably happy doing what only women of low character were suppose to do. When she pleaded with her parents to set her free of social obligations to study nursing at The Institution of Kaiserswerth, one of the best teaching hospitals in Europe, her mother accused her of conducting a secret love affair with a "low vulgar surgeon," and would not hear of it. Her sister fainted at the mere mention of such a plan (who would marry a sister of a woman like that?). Her father took off to the spas in Baden-Baden and would not even discuss such madness.

At twenty-six, Florence collapsed into hopeless depression. Light gave her headaches, noise made her jumpy, her mind wandered perpetually into what she described as "dreaming," and for eight years she was to all outward appearances a curious invalid. Although her family did not wish her to suffer, they were content enough with Florence's situation not to look for a real cure. Her headaches were treated with narcotics and calming work about the house. (Her mother put her in charge of managing the estate's pantry and linen closets.) Long stays in the country, away from the excitement of London, and slow travel to distant lands were also recommended. Such were the strong restrictions of her class that it took an ill-advised and bloody war to rouse Nightingale from what would otherwise have been a life of quiet desperation. From November 5, 1854, when she first stepped into the British army's hospital in Scutari, Turkey, to July 16, 1856, when the last of the wounded and sick were sent back home, Nightingale slaved and fought—against obstinate, imperious physicians and callous officials—to improve the conditions of the wounded soldiers. Some of the improvements she made were simple and now seem commonsensi-cal (bed linens changed daily, clean shirts for the patients, properly ventilated wards), others were revolutionary for their time (adequate and nutritious meals for every patient—even the most common-born soldier—hospital buildings constructed away from city sewers and cemeteries). In less than two years, she transformed the idea of caring for the sick from a haphazard, often futile and filthy chore where the best that could be offered was a small degree of comfort, to a precise practice that could actually save lives.

While it's true that, if she lived today, Florence would have had a much easier—and straighter—road to travel toward her life's goal, I sometimes think that certain situations have not changed. Women continue to lead oblique lives, impelled to carry on many different—sometimes warring—obligations between accomplishing their desires and playing the roles society continues to expect of them. I first be-came aware of this situation when, shortly out of college and liv-ing far away on my own, I came down with a sudden illness whose strongest symptom was periods of debilitating headaches. I could not lift my head, could not move even a toe without a jolt of blinding pain shuddering through my body. There was a very high fever on the first day, then nothing except the headaches. I lay on my narrow bed in my small room watching through slitted eyes as the leaves on the enormous trees outside my windows gradually changed colors through the balmy southern autumn. Friends would drop by to see me, take one look at my pale face, and beg me to see a doctor. I think now that the sight of someone their own age so enfeebled must have frightened them. But I don't remember being concerned at all—a little annoyed, perhaps, by the constraints on my social life but more often amused by the foolish postures the pain forced me into. I read with my head tilted sideways cradled in a mass of pillows; walked to the bathroom bracing my face between my hands as if I was holding a fragile custard. It was not at all unpleasant to lie in that room, which seemed to nestle coolly in the upper canopy of the surrounding oak trees. I was enveloped by time, good books, and music, with an excellent excuse to be away from a terrible job. The truth, perhaps, was that I knew I was drifting in my convalescent contentment, using the illness to bide my time while one life blurred and another all too slowly came into focus.

I would have happily loitered in my bed for some time if a rather imperious man I still can't believe I got myself involved with hadn't taken hold of the situation and made an appointment with a man he assured me was one of the best doctors in Atlanta. The doctor was associated with the government, and since my job was under contract with the state, all his enormous bills would be duly paid without question. The next day, my friend drove me to the office in a fashionable suburb. When it was my turn to see the doctor, I forced my friend to remain in the waiting room and walked in to meet a nice-looking, middle-aged man with courtly manners. The doctor listened to my story, took a few notes, then outlined a battery of tests for the next few days that would leave no part of my body untouched. I meekly submitted to a few that day in his office that weren't too bad—a thorough examination and a complete recording of my vital signs. The next day I endured a C.A.T. scan, some kind of eye test involving a laser, and, toward the end of the day, when I truly had a headache, a couple of psychological tests that were beginning to raise warning signs. But at a time when I was still in awe of anyone who was supposed to be my superior, it did not occur to me to protest at all. Back in his office, after I listened to the next day's program, which involved inserting tubes in places I knew had nothing to do with my head, I asked the doctor what he thought the results of all this would be. He smiled rather patiently at me from across his desk and said, "It's hard to tell. With women and Negroes, you have to take into account other things."

Like what, I inquired, really curious—if not downright obtuse—about what he could be getting at.

"Well," he sighed. "Sometimes, unfortunately, it's a lack of formal education but mostly it's just the general weakness in inferior constitutions."

I didn't even thank him for his time. I banged open the office door, sailed past my friend, and never went back again, the doctor's exorbitant bill for services rendered never submitted for payment. The headaches slowly disappeared. I am now convinced that they were the product of a low-grade infection that would have been properly considered had I been a man. Soon afterward, at our last meeting, when I was breaking things off with him, my friend informed me that the doctor had warned him I was a classic hysteric and advised him not to become seriously involved with me.

"Then you shouldn't mind," I replied and, not as casually as I had wished, walked away.

I NEVER MET another doctor quite so blatant in his prejudices, and yet I remain a little skeptical about doctors in general (though I have nothing but strong faith in our current doctor, who has seen my family through various crises in fine, intelligent style). I have heard enough tales from other women to be convinced that women are still viewed somewhat differently from men when it comes to their ailments. The stories women tell about their experiences with doctors are usually related with indignation, even horror, yet they continue to chalk up these transgressions to a lot of things that should not be forgiven.

I don't see any reason in the world to suffer a fool, especially when my health is at stake. Yet, as I think about the matter, I am not unwilling to consider the fact that the situation may have something to do with the intricacies of a woman's body. Without the complications associated with reproduction, men's operating systems are, by comparison, straightforward. What goes wrong with them is usually clearer than what can go haywire in women. And because men have a soldier-like reputation, their complaints are often considered to be grounded in reality. As a result, I have very rarely heard anything but praise from men about their doctors and the cures they prescribed for them. (Now, you ask any woman who's ever lived with a man if this is true in an informal, away-from-the-doctor's-office way, and she'll just laugh at you. The term "baby," often with the adjective "big" before it, is not an uncommon opinion about the supposed stoicism of men.)

But for everyone—male and female alike—(and I suspect this has always been so, even in the paternalistic shelter of the nineteenth century), it is often the case that what really ails us is only remotely related to anything a doctor may have studied in school. This is no truer than when a good old-fashioned headache, whose source is not remotely physiological, strikes.

In my case, I know it's often because my days start early and go on sometimes to midnight, followed frequently by fitful sleep. I deal with a job that is always nerve-racking, navigate my children through dangerous periods in their lives, strive with all my heart to continue a marriage that is like most—almost always a passionate refuge but not infrequently a maddening entanglement. In between, there are warring forces of good and evil—ill-tempered bosses, aggravating parents, unpaid bills, leaking roofs, neighbors with deafening stereo speakers. No wonder, then, that during some part of these many hours, I develop a headache or, on really bad days, feel like pulling a Nightingale and taking to my bed. The only thing that has stopped me from this course is the realization that, as a member of a poorer class, I would not have the luxury of being tended to as Florence was. No one would coddle me. No one would whisk me away to a palazzo on the Grand Canal.

What I do instead is to look for the cause and try to alleviate it as best I can, helping it along with a little medicinal sustenance. The most common causes of headaches are stress—in daily life or from the wear of illnesses; environmental factors (like pollen and pollution resulting in allergies and sinus pressure); or by-products of something else going on with the body (fevers, menstruation, hunger, hangovers, fatigue). If headaches become frequent or are debilitating, they should be carefully explored. There are now a wonderful array of treatment options, from new prescriptive medicines to alternative methods such as acupuncture, pain management therapy, and herbal preparations. Migraines are in a class by themselves, and must be treated under a competent doctor's care.

But simple headaches can be easily managed, especially these days, with the miracle of aspirin and other over-the-counter aids. For added potency, I combine two aspirins with one of the following old remedies. Teas in particular are a favorite cure, perhaps because the directions are always emphatic about sipping them while lying down. I brew the potion and carry the cup to the sofa or, if the headache is really bad, to my bedroom, where I close the door. Propped up among the pillows on the bed, I swallow the aspirins and slowly sip the brew, sometimes falling off into a refreshing sleep, but most times just benefiting from the exquisite pause in the day.

VERVAIN TEA

Makes 1 serving

In the old cookbook in which I found this tea (*Directions for Cookery* by Miss Eliza Leslie, 1828), an accompanying note stresses that it is beneficial to excitable young ladies and tired nursing mothers.

1 cup fresh blue verbena leaves and flowers, finely chopped

Honey to taste

Add 2 teaspoons chopped leaves and flowers to 2 cups boiling water.

Sip while lying down.

Note: The original recipe doesn't say, but you can dry the remaining leaves and flowers and store in an airtight bottle.

CATNIP TEA

Makes 1 serving

This is an old Amish tea recipe for people, which also works well for ill-tempered cats.

1 young catnip plant	Strip plant of its leaves. Break the twigs into several pieces. (A young plant should yield about 2 cups of leaves and twigs.) Place in a small saucepan with 1 cup of water and bring to a boil. Turn off the heat and let steep for 5 minutes. Strain. Sip the liquid slowly while lying down in a darkened room.

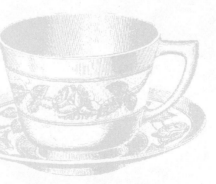

HERB TEA FOR HEADACHES

Makes enough for 1 pot of tea, about 4 servings

Several other herbs, such as sage, balm (lemon balm is a delicious choice), rosemary, and southerwood are excellent for headaches when steeped as teas. You should gather the leaves on summer mornings when they are young, then dry them and seal the crumbled leaves in an airtight container or bag for use throughout the year. You'll find these herbs have a grassy taste, with a heavy oily feel that lingers in the throat. Sipping this tea is as pleasant as lying under a summer quilt.

¼ cup leaves from a young plant (suggested plants listed above)

2 tablespoons sugar

Zest from 1 lemon

Thoroughly clean the leaves, being careful not to bruise them, which would rob them of juice. Place the leaves, sugar, and lemon zest in 2 pints boiling water in a saucepan, turn off the heat under the pan, and let steep for 1 hour.

Strain the ingredients through a fine-mesh sieve. Reheat the liquid until it's hot. Serve immediately, making sure the patient sips slowly.

ROSE TEA

Makes enough for 1 pot of tea, about 4 servings

This tea is very pretty. It was recommended by Dr. Robert Wallace Johnson in *The Nurse's Guide* (1819) for summer headaches, sunstrokes, and general overexhaustion. If there is any tea left over, he suggests soaking a fine linen handkerchief in it and applying it to the forehead, then resting, with eyes closed, in the cool shadows of a shade tree.

½ cup red rosebuds, white heel removed

3 teaspoons wine vinegar

2 tablespoons sugar

Place the rosebuds, vinegar, and sugar in a medium saucepan and cover with 2 pints boiling water. Let steep for 2 hours.

Strain through a fine mesh and serve warm, not hot.

LAVENDER COMPOUND

Makes about 1 quart—usually about a year's supply

This lavender mixture is not a tea but it is very potent. Ladies used to carry small vials of it in their purses when they went to social gatherings and pressed small dabs of it to their temples and pulse points to calm their nerves. For modern times, use it in a similar manner to reduce stress, lying with eyes closed for a few minutes before resuming activity. To use as a headache cure: Pour a small amount over a sugar cube and place the cube on your tongue. Let it dissolve slowly. Take as necessary.

1   cup freshly
    gathered lavender
    blossoms
1   quart very good
    brandy
1   tablespoon each
    clove, mace,
    nutmeg

Loosely fill a glass quart bottle with the lavender blossoms. Pour in the brandy to cover and put a stopper in the bottle. Let stand a fortnight (14 days).

Uncork the bottle and add the clove, mace, and nutmeg. Cork the bottle and shake vigorously. Pour the liquid off into smaller glass bottles or vials and cork them. May be used immediately.

PEPPERMINT EGG SOUP

Makes 6 small servings

Peppermint was considered a very good cure for headaches of all kinds, especially those associated with overactivity. The leaves were chewed raw or steeped as tea, but this soup, I think, is a steadier application. It comes from Mary Boland Pequignot's *A Handbook of Invalid Cooking* (1893) and she recommends it, rather pointedly, for what she refers to as "overindulgence," meaning a hangover. This does not keep well—a day at best.

1 bunch (about 1 full cup) young fresh peppermint leaves, washed and picked over

1 large egg per serving

In a medium saucepan, bring 1 quart water to a boil and add the peppermint leaves. Cook at a very slow simmer for 5 minutes. Remove from the heat.

Measure about 1 cup per serving and heat slowly to a boil in a small saucepan. Add an egg and poach it gently in the liquid until the desired consistency is reached. Pour into small bowl and serve at once. Repeat the poaching procedure as additional servings are needed.

BUTTERMILK PAP

Makes 1 serving

Here's another hangover cure that works on a sour stomach as well as an aching head. It's a folk remedy offered by my neighbor, Earl, an exceedingly tall, stout Norwegian who used to work the Brooklyn docks in the 1920s. He remembers his mother giving it to him the first time he came home drunk. He was sixteen and it was after his first paycheck. The men took him out to a local bar and got him so drunk they tied a rope around his waist and threw him into the river, then fished him out and pushed him back home, dragging him up the steep brownstone steps and into his mother's arms. At ninety-two, Earl's eyes are cloudy, half blind with cataracts. But he looked at me with an unwavering sharpness and grabbed my arm as he leaned forward on the same stoop he was carted up that day and laughed, "After I drank all what she gave me down, I got a lickin' with a cat-o'-nine-tails and never told her about another hangover again."

1 tablespoon cornstarch

1 cup good fresh buttermilk

Salt and pepper

Mix the cornstarch with the buttermilk and heat gently in a medium saucepan. Do not boil! Cook until just heated through.

Add a little salt and pepper to taste and sip like soup while it's hot. Or you can cool it slightly, stir in a lot of honey, and pour it into a tall glass to sip slowly through the day.

◄§ TREATMENT FOR §► NYMPHOMANIA

(This recipe is included for its historical relevance only.
*It is **not** recommended for modern-day use.)*

Overexertion of any kind was a cause of alarm in the nineteenth century and none more so than when a young woman became what in polite circles was referred to as "restless." This was often a code word for sexually active, a state of affairs that was unfortunate in any case but particularly distressing when the patient came from a good Christian family. How did such a disease occur? The editors of the textbook, *Sexual Ills and Diseases* (1896), recorded a case—one they said was becoming all too familiar—of a twenty-three-year-old woman whose parents foolishly allowed her not only to attend college (Bryn Mawr), but to travel extensively in Europe on her own, without a chaperone. When she returned to take up her duties in her family home outside of Philadelphia, it was discovered that she was not only unhappy with helping her mother but also spending far too much time with certain men. She was found to be unmarriageable and increasingly unmanageable. Here is the treatment outlined for her:

In order of preference and effectiveness, have the patient partake first of cannabis, steeped in tea, to be consumed every four hours over the course of one month.

If improvement is not noted, consider adding to this regime: *Cimicifuga racemosa* (black cohosh, an herb popularly used as an antidote against poisons and snakebites) taken as a tea, or coffee (black and strong); or in the worst cases, and as a last resort, *Erythroxylum coca* (cocaine) in powdered form, diluted with water.

Contending with the Vapors

Fainting, especially among women, was once far more prevalent than it is today. There was even a special piece of furniture to swoon upon, called a fainting couch, which was very popular in the early 1800s. (It is the delicately framed chaise longue across which Ingres' odalisques stretch languorously.) The general cause of fainting, in the opinion of Dr. Johnson and Dr. John Fothergill of the London Society of Physicians, was fashion. The main culprits were stays and corsets which produced the small waists in favor through most of the nineteenth century. In *The Nurse's Guide,* Dr. Johnson warned pregnant women not to wear any form of restraints, lest the baby be born deformed. He also thought that young girls should not be bound until at least the age of fifteen, "though modern modesty—and the marriage market—may dictate otherwise," he lamented. The constraints corsets put on the lungs curtailed breathing and compromised the stomach in digesting food. Even robust, healthy women regularly fainted and always carried about assorted remedies to alleviate the lesser symptoms of light-headedness and dizziness.

A friend of mine who makes her living writing for magazines recently fell under the sway of corsets after writing an article about them for a fetish magazine. She is a very beautiful, athletic woman and, tightly laced in the boned silk cage, her already fine figure blossomed into such a strangely alluring shape that she began to wear the thing to all the parties and dinners she attended. Of strong Midwestern stock, Kathleen's been sick only once in her adult life and that was a minor cold that lasted two weeks just like everyone else's. But when she wore the corset she reported that there were times when she felt her breathing become so shallow that she'd have to lean upon the arm of any soul conveniently nearby. Most times it was a man, and though at first she enjoyed the attention, she soon grew weary of its implications. She could eat only very small portions before she began to feel nausea, and any activity beyond walking caused her to lose her breath. Off went the corset and the poor men it had lured were mightily surprised when she emerged from its constraints as the rather steely force of nature she usually is.

I have never been given to fainting, no matter what the circumstances, but I have seen it several times in people I love when they've been gravely ill or are on a foolishly rigorous diet. In the latter case, salted crackers or small pieces of a good yeasty bread are beneficial, followed by a stern lecture on being more level-headed about losing weight. When someone is feeling faint as a result of illness, check to see how high her fever is and if she's taking enough liquids. A high fever will produce light-headedness and the body needs fluids to cool itself down.

ALBUMENIZED MILK

Makes 1 serving

Dr. James W. Allan, the superintendent of the City of Glasgow's Fever Hospital, recommended in his small book, *Notes on Fever Nursing* (1880), that his patients be given small quantities of slightly chilled milk until the fever subsided. A good recipe is this one for albumenized milk, which comes from *The Rumford Complete Cook Book* (1908).

1 large egg white (powdered egg white may be substituted, or use the directions on page 14 to cook)

¼ cup seltzer

1 cup cold milk

Place all the ingredients in a blender and mix to blend. Strain and serve at once, as is or sweetened with a little honey or sugar.

. . .

DR. WILLIAM W. HALL was a very popular author/doctor in the late 1800s, publishing a series of books on contemporary health hazards. He recommended rubbing the feet of fever patients with a sliced onion in his book, *Health by Good Living* (1870). The onion, he said, will turn black, signifying that it is drawing all the offending noxious poisons from the body.

WATERMELON FOR FEVERS

Makes 1 serving

A better recommendation is his suggestion to eat watermelon. The following recipe is beneficial for two reasons: It is cold and will help draw heat away from the body, and it is full of liquid to replace what is probably being lost through sweating.

1 large slice of ripe watermelon	Slice the flesh of the melon into small, bite-size cubes. Remove all the seeds. Place the pieces in a glass or china bowl and chill thoroughly.
	To serve, add cracked ice and a little water (about 2 tablespoons) to slightly dilute the watermelon juice. Have the patient eat as much of the melon as he can, but in particular, have him drink—or slowly sip—the juice. Repeat as necessary.

THE EMPERIAL DRINK

Makes 4 to 6 servings

Dr. Robert Wallace Johnson ordered this rather grandly named drink to be made in quantities at parties as a precautionary measure when the excitement of dancing proved overwhelming. It is, despite the presence of barley water, a tasty drink, very good for fevers that are accompanied by sour stomachs. Barley water is made by combining fine-grain pearl barley (sold in specialty stores) with water and lemon (see page 76).

½ teaspoon cream of tartar

Zest from 1 lemon or 1 orange, pith removed

3 tablespoons sugar

2 pints barley water

Combine all the ingredients in a stone or porcelain jug and refrigerate for 10 minutes. Strain and serve.

. . .

I HAVE TWO MORE remedies that are meant to revive the spirit when it's been wilted by a strong fever or the demands of the day.

ORANGE GELATIN DRINK

Makes 1 serving

This first may be given during the course of the fever to help cool down the body and calm jittery nerves. Just be certain that the stomach is not unduly troubled, because orange juice is very acidic and may cause stomach upset. The drink should be sipped or spooned very slowly.

1 packet unflavored gelatin

1 cup freshly squeezed orange juice

In a medium bowl, mix the gelatin with 2 tablespoons cold water. Add the orange juice and stir well until the gelatin is dissolved. Refrigerate until *only* partially set and serve cool (not cold, which could further upset a delicate stomach).

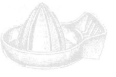

COCOA CORDIAL

Makes 1 serving

I have found this final drink, from Fannie Farmer's *Food and Cookery for the Sick and Convalescent* (1904), to be of great benefit when taken in the late afternoon—a time of day when most people, no matter if they are sick or well, are feeling a little jagged. I have given it to my husband when his spirits were sagging after a small illness; I last served it to my mother when she was recuperating from throat cancer and the diminishing afternoon light filtering through her room made her a bit forlorn. And I often make this for myself, when my children are clamoring for more than I can give them, when the demands of the world are all too great—when the source of all the tremors in my head and soul will not be found in medical journals but in the simple script of daily life.

1 teaspoon Dutch-process cocoa

1 teaspoon sugar

1½ to 3 tablespoons best quality port wine (depending on the state of your nerves)

Mix together the cocoa and sugar in a medium saucepan. Boil ½ cup water and add just enough to form a paste. Stir in the remaining water and bring to a boil for 1 minute. Remove from heat and pour into a mug. Add port wine. (In case of a bad day, add more wine.)

Honking and Wheezing

Colds and Coughs

Giving into a cold used to be a fine excuse for bringing life to a halt. Not at death's door, but enough to justify remaining in bed, apologies were made and sympathetically accepted. The sufferer was then allowed to wallow, free of guilt, in contented misery.

How civilized! And how hard, in contrast, seems modern life with its quick prescriptions and convenient bromides readily available on drugstore shelves to make it all but impossible to go into seclusion. Antibiotics have saved susceptible young children and old people from succumbing to complications. There are shelves of drugs to get us easily through the more minor discomforts of sinus headaches, runny noses, and scratchy throats. So a cold or cough, even the flu, is easy to dismiss with a few pills. Life is expected to go on, no matter how befuddled the brain or how aching the body.

. . .

AND YET IT IS BETTER, I think, to resort to the prescription a friend of mine passed on to me when she came back from living for many years in New Orleans. She had gone there with her two young daughters in the hope of recovering from a painful divorce and with the offer of a very good job. New Orleans seemed perfect to her at first; the weather, when she arrived in spring and even through a simmering summer, pleasantly suited her northern bones and she fell in love with the city's architecture, in particular the old house she rented in one of the outlying parishes. But the autumn turned unusually chilly, underlined by a dampness that left nothing dry for long. By the first of an icy December, the walls on the first floor of the house wore specks of green mildew, and she and the girls were miserable with lingering colds. The house, she wrote, sounded like a coffin ship at night with all the hacking; her daughters were visibly fading before her eyes. Finally, a neighbor woman stepped in. She put them all to bed and dished out small bowls of Lait de Poule, a restorative soup of egg, milk, and broth her French ancestors have sworn by for centuries to cure colds. A week of bed rest, the warming soup (and a new heating system for the house), and they were on their way. My friend was behind in work. The children had to make up their school lessons. But they were so much better.

LAIT DE POULE

Makes 6 small servings

1 large egg yolk
½ cup milk or cream
2 cups beef, chicken, or vegetable broth

Add the yolk to the milk in a medium bowl and beat well until slightly frothy. Heat the broth to a simmer, then add the yolk mixture, stirring with a wooden spoon. Cook until the egg is set into soft curds. Serve at once.

A NOURISHING CHICKEN BROTH

Makes about six 1-cup servings

One of the reasons soups are so good for a cold is that the warm liquid helps stimulate secretions and unclogs stuffed nasal passages. Chicken soup, of course, has a long history of curing colds. The medical proof is skimpy, to be sure, but people have sworn by its powers for generations. A very good—and potent—recipe is found in Fannie Farmer's *Food and Cookery for the Sick and Convalescent* (1904).

2   veal knuckles
    (about 2 pounds)
1   whole chicken
    carcass, stripped of
    meat, bones
    cracked open (to
    give access to the
    nutritious marrow)
1   ham bone (about 2
    pounds)
6   carrots, peeled and
    sliced in thin
    rounds
2   celery stalks, sliced
½   bay leaf
¼   teaspoon
    peppercorns
1   medium onion,
    minced
2   smashed eggshells

Put all the bones in a large stockpot and cover with water. Bring to a boil, then lower the heat and simmer for 4 or 5 hours, skimming the scum that will rise to the top. Remove the bones, then strain the liquid into a bowl through layers of cheesecloth.

Wipe out the stockpot and return the liquid to the pot by straining it again through a sieve lined with cheesecloth. Add the carrots, celery, bay leaf, peppercorns, onion, and eggshells.

Bring the mixture to a rolling simmer and cook until the vegetables are soft. Again strain, this time using a fine-mesh strainer and pushing the vegetables and eggshells against the mesh with the back of a wooden spoon to remove all the essence. Discard the vegetables and eggshells and serve only the broth.

QUEEN VICTORIA'S FAVORITE SOUP

Makes 4 servings

The chicken soup Queen Victoria made is a delicate, filling concoction. It is recorded in Mary Boland Pequignot's book, *A Handbook of Invalid Cooking* (1893), which notes that the queen made it often for her husband and children at their country home. (I like to think of her sneaking down in the middle of the night when the servants were in bed and making the soup like the middle-class housewife she seems to have been at heart.)

½ cup oyster cracker crumbs or fresh bread crumbs

1 pint sweet cream

1 pint *very* strong fresh chicken broth

1 cup chopped raw chicken breast

3 hard-cooked large egg yolks

Salt and freshly ground pepper

Soak the crumbs in 1 cup of the cream until soft. Meanwhile, bring the broth to a boil in a stainless steel pot and add the chopped chicken. Simmer gently to cook the chicken until the meat is very soft. Then stir the cream and crumb mixture into the broth.

Press the yolks through a fine sieve into the broth. Add salt and pepper to taste. Strain the broth through a colander, pressing on the chicken and crumbs with the back of a wooden spoon. Return the strained broth to the pot. Add the remaining 1 cup of cream a little at a time, stirring gently, and bring to a boil. Simmer for 5 minutes to heat through.

SCUTARI BROTH

Makes 4 servings

A good broth for invalids was recommended by Alexis Soyer in his book, *The Modern Housewife* (1859). Soyer was a renowned chef in London when he volunteered to help Florence Nightingale in the Crimea—an event that in its day would be akin to David Bouley signing up for kitchen duty during the Persian Gulf War. Soyer joined Nightingale, whom he called the "genteel Amazone," at the Barrack Hospital at Scutari, Turkey, to improve the diet of the wounded soldiers, and after the war to reform the design of the army's field kitchens. In the hospital, faced with wards packed with men suffering from every sort of disease and injury, one of the first things he made was a veal broth that French doctors recommended to quell night coughs. Nightingale instructed that the ingredients be procured (cabbage and chervil being hard to find during the Turkish winter) and great pots of the soup—enough to truly feed an army—were immediately brewed. I have modified his recipe for smaller quantities.

1 pound cracked marrow veal bones	In a large soup pot, bring the veal bones and 6 cups water to a boil. Skim the scum that will rise to the top. Reduce the heat, cover, and simmer for 3 to 4 hours, adding more water as needed.
1 small green cabbage, stripped of tough outer leaves and chopped	
3 chervil sprigs	Add the cabbage leaves and chervil.

> Simmer for ½ hour more. Discard the veal
> bones and strain through a fine sieve, pressing
> cabbage and chervil leaves against the side of
> the sieve to press out all liquid. Discard leaves.
> Serve broth warm, not hot.

Note: Soyer notes in his book that, for civilians, this recipe can be refined by adding I teaspoon sweet butter; ½ medium onion, chopped; I carrot, chopped; I turnip, chopped; and 2 celery stalks, chopped.

Return broth to a simmer and add these ingredients. Cook slowly at a simmer until the vegetables are tender, about 20 minutes. For an even heartier soup, a handful of vermicelli can be added during the last few minutes. Serve with the vegetables in the broth.

SAFFRON CONSOMMÉ

Makes 6 servings

My own favorite broth is not an old recipe. I found it in a copy of *The Pleasures of Cooking* several years ago. It's a saffron consommé whose rich smell (provided you can still smell through a clogged nose) is surely half the cure.

Start this recipe by making the white stock and skim as much grease as you can from it. It helps to let the stock sit overnight in the refrigerator.

WHITE STOCK

5 pounds veal bones (including a knuckle), cracked

2 pounds chicken parts (backs, wings, or necks)

1 pound stewing veal, cut into 2-inch cubes

1 large carrot, cut into 1-inch pieces

1 celery stalk with top, cut into 1-inch pieces

To make the stock, put the veal bones, chicken parts, and stewing veal into a large stockpot and add enough water to cover by 2 inches. Bring to a boil, reduce the heat, and simmer, uncovered, for 5 minutes.

Drain and rinse the bones and meat under cold water to remove all the scum. Rinse and wipe the inside of the stockpot.

Return the meat and bones to the stockpot and add 3 quarts of water. Bring to a boil over high heat, skimming often. Add the carrot, celery, leek, onion, parsley,

1 medium leek, white and tender green part only, thoroughly washed and cut into 1-inch pieces

1 onion, peeled and halved

6 parsley sprigs

2 teaspoons kosher salt

Freshly ground pepper

salt, and pepper to taste. Reduce the heat, partially cover, and simmer gently for about 3 hours, skimming occasionally.

Strain the stock through a double layer of cheesecloth, discarding the solids. The stock keeps, covered and refrigerated, for 3 or 4 days; or it can be frozen for up to 6 months. Skim the fat from the surface before using.

CONSOMMÉ

2 tablespoons grated onion

6 cups white stock, chilled and thoroughly degreased

2 large egg whites

2 eggshells, crushed

½ teaspoon saffron threads or ¼ teaspoon ground saffron

Salt and freshly ground pepper

Make the consommé: Place the grated onion in a fine sieve over a small bowl and press down on it with the back of a spoon to extract the juices. Measure and set aside I teaspoon of the onion juice. Discard the rest.

Bring the stock to a boil over high heat in a large saucepan. Meanwhile, whisk the egg whites in a small bowl until frothy. When the stock is boiling, stir in the egg whites and eggshells, reduce the heat, and simmer gently, without stirring, for about 20 minutes. Strain the stock into a slightly smaller stockpot through a large sieve lined with several thicknesses of rinsed cheesecloth. Bring to a simmer over moderate heat and stir in the reserved onion juice.

If you are using saffron threads, crush them between your fingers and place in a small dish. Add about ¼ cup of the hot stock, stir gently to dissolve the saffron, then pour the mixture into the simmering stock. If you are using ground saffron, whisk directly into the simmering stock. Simmer for 3 to 5 minutes more to let the flavor develop. Add salt and pepper to taste.

SWEET LAIT DE POULE

Makes 2 servings

Another French cure from my friend in New Orleans is made from orange flower water, a perfumey flavoring you can find in baking shops and gourmet stores. The accompanying note from the old woman who gave this recipe to my friend reads, "Drink this very hot while lying still in bed, the head and shoulders propped up by many plump pillows; I can strongly recommend it from experience." It is beneficial for sore throats.

2   large egg yolks

2   teaspoons sugar

4   drops orange flower water (can substitute ⅛ teaspoon finely grated lemon zest)

Beat the yolks with the sugar and orange flower water in a saucepan until they're nicely frothy. Place the saucepan over low heat and cook the yolk mixture, stirring constantly, until it coats a wooden spoon with a thin film, or the temperature reaches 160°F.

Pour the yolk mixture into a mug or teacup and gradually add about 1 cup boiling water, stirring constantly, until the cup is full.

BLACK CURRANT TEA

Makes 1 serving

Teas and other warm beverages are also recommended for colds and coughs. My husband's grandmother used to make his mother black currant tea whenever she had a cold. Doris was in no way a particularly maternal woman. In fact, she was one of the vainest, most mean-spirited people I have ever met, who, nevertheless, loved Chris's mom to a fault. She was a working-class German Protestant girl who married an up-and-coming man of Jewish heritage because, she was wont to say in plain hearing of everyone (including her husband and his relatives), the Jews possessed great genes and she wanted her children to be smart and ambitious. It also helped that the man she picked was on his way to making a tidy fortune in real estate. I don't know if Doris cooked. There certainly are no family stories or even memories of her doing so, but this one recipe was told to me by Chris's mom with a deep longing for the comfort she received from it, perhaps because it was one of the very few times she was allowed to nestle in her mother's lap.

2 tablespoons good-quality black currant jam	Spoon the jam into a large teacup or mug. Pour 1 cup boiling water over it and stir until the jam is dissolved. Drink it all while it's still hot.

HOT LEMONADE

Makes 1 serving

Another good hot fruity drink is hot lemonade. The following recipe is from *The Rumford Complete Cook Book* (1908).

2 or 3 lumps of sugar 1 large lemon	Rub the sugar over the outside of the lemon to extract a little of the flavor, then dust it off into a teacup, adding any leftover sugar. Cut the lemon in half and squeeze the juice into the cup over the sugar. Stir until the sugar is dissolved. Add about 1 cup boiling water and stir again. Float a slice of lemon in the liquid for added potency.

Note: I often substitute 1 heaping tablespoon honey for the sugar and, of course, omit rubbing it over the lemon skin unless you like the goo. If I am truly suffering and ready to go to bed, I might do as my mother would: I'd also add what she would call a "nip" of whiskey. That translates into about a shot and a half of liquor. Brandy also does nicely.

ICELAND LEMONADE

Makes about 6 servings

A final lemonade recipe comes from *Common Sense in the Household* by Marion Harland (originally published in 1871 under her real name, Mary Virginia Hawes Terhune, and continually revised until 1926). This book is a cross between *Joy of Cooking* and *Hints from Heloise* (a rather grumpy Heloise, at that) but it is full of good insights into nineteenth-century middle-class American sensibilities. While making a pretty good living as a writer, Mrs. Harland espoused the belief that a woman's place was ordained by sacred orders to remain firmly in the home. She was also something of a Nativist and was appalled by the influx of immigrants coming into the country. The paragraph before she gives this recipe talks about the importance of not looking like "a common Irish girl," "with your hair at odds and ends, smelling of the kitchen, when you bring this to your poor husband or babes." The main ingredient in this recipe is Irish moss—seaweed—and can be found in health food stores. This beverage is slippery on the throat, full of vitamins, and very bracing. It is recommended for feverish colds and all pulmonary discomforts.

1 handful (about
½ cup) Irish moss

2 medium lemons,
peeled and sliced
in thin rounds

Honey or sugar

Wash the moss under a steady stream of water until all the sand is removed. Place the moss in a glass pitcher and pour 2 quarts boiling water over it. Add the lemon slices and let steep for at least an hour, stirring occasionally.

To serve, strain the liquid through a fine mesh and pour over cracked ice. Add honey or sugar to taste.

. . .

VINEGAR IS USUALLY recommended to clean out the intestines, but I've found several vinegar drinks specifically for colds. The astringency is believed to cut through phlegm and mucus, clearing the head and lungs.

The most agreeable I've found is from Alexis Soyer, who claimed he found it of great use not just for colds but also in helping with scurvy and, when used externally, to lower the temperature of feverish patients (by rubbing the patient's body down with it, then placing a cloth soaked in the mixture across the forehead). A simple drink to do all that but, nevertheless, pleasant.

A RASPBERRY CURE

Makes about 4 servings

2 tablespoons
   raspberry vinegar

Place the vinegar and 1 cup boiling water in a cup and stir to blend. Sip warm for colds. For fevers, chill the liquid, soak a cloth in it,then press the cloth against the forehead, underarms, and extremities. Repeat as necessary until fever falls.

. . .

LESS AGREEABLE, to me at least, and yet sworn by in not one but three old books for invalids, is a cold vinegar drink. M. F. K. Fisher even mentions it in *A Cordiall Water,* as favored by a famous Methodist preacher, Peter Cartwright, who took it every time his throat became raw from spreading the good word across the Midwestern religious circuit in the latter part of the nineteenth century. I first came across it in Dr. Robert Wallace Johnson's *The Nurse's Guide,* then stumbled upon it again in the very sensible Mary Boland Pequignot's *A Handbook of Invalid Cooking.* The final place I found it was in *The Rumford Complete Cook Book.* I've recorded Mrs. Pequignot's recipe because her measurements are so exact and, as the head nurse at Johns Hopkins University, she seems to be a trustworthy soul.

A VINEGAR DRINK FOR COLDS

Makes 1 serving

Let me be frank about this recipe: The heat of the pepper will very nearly kill you. On the first sip, the mouth twists into a gasp and a hoarse rasp bellows involuntarily from the throat. The recommendation is to drink the entire glass in one sitting, as painful as it may seem. I can report that it works. My chest and throat burned with a hard (yet not altogether unpleasant) heat but subsided into a banked warmth. The soreness in my throat was, indeed, gone. So was any feeling or taste sensation in my mouth. As an extra bonus, my nasal passages cleared. It's hard to advocate such a slash and burn cure but there is a reason why it's been recorded—and handed down—so faithfully over these many years.

½ cup icy cold good quality white wine vinegar 1 teaspoon salt ½ teaspoon (!) cayenne pepper	Stir all the ingredients together in a tall glass until the salt and cayenne dissolve. Let the drink warm to room temperature, then stir once more and refrigerate until thoroughly chilled again. Serve cold and sip gradually.

SWEET CIDER SYRUP

Makes 1 serving

A far more agreeable cider preparation is one made from sweet apple cider, prescribed by Dr. William Hall.

1 cup sweet apple cider	Place the cider in a stainless steel saucepan and bring to a gentle boil. Let simmer until the liquid is reduced by half. Drink warm or cold.

. . .

THE FOLLOWING cough remedies may seem worse than the symptoms but they do work. The most potent is one made from the bark of the North American slippery elm tree (also known as red elm). It uses only the inner bark. Instead of going on a search through the woods, find instead a very good health food store.

SLIPPERY ELM BARK TEA

Makes 1 day's serving

This particular recipe comes from the Mohawk Indians; with small variations, I have also seen it recorded in Marion Harland's *Common Sense in the Household* (though I'm inclined to think she would not admit to any such heathen lineage). Harland suggests the addition of lemon slices, which takes a little of the earthiness off the flavor, but not by much.

One 2-inch piece of
    slippery elm bark,
    broken into pieces
⅛ teaspoon cayenne
    pepper

Place the bark in a jug and add the cayenne and 2 cups boiling water to it. Let it stand for 25 minutes. Take this frequently in small doses. Patients with very bad, persistent coughs should consume about a pint a day.

PECTORIAL   DRINK

Makes 1 quart

I found this useful expectorant in Dr. Robert Wallace Johnson's book.

1 tablespoon pearl
   barley
1 tablespoon raisins
½ tablespoon licorice

Bring 2 quarts water to a boil in a large
saucepan, then add the barley, raisins, and
licorice. Stir to mix and continue to simmer
until reduced by half (it will get thick).
Remove from the heat and let cool. Serve
warm or cool. Take it a teaspoon at a time,
as needed.

. . .

THE NEXT THREE preparations are a little more disagreeable. The
first is based on oatmeal and the others on vegetables, in this case an
onion and a turnip. In each you use the juice produced by the recipe.
They are all specified for coughs.

OATMEAL BROSE

Makes about 1 cup

1 cup oats (the long-simmering kind)

Pinch of salt

1 tablespoon butter

1 tablespoon sugar

Put the oatmeal in a bowl with the salt, butter, and sugar. Pour on 2 cups boiling water, stirring all the time.

Let the oatmeal steep for a minute, then pour into a fine mesh sieve and let the liquid drain into a container with a lid. Discard the oatmeal. Drink the liquid hot or at room temperature (but it tastes better if it's heated a little) at bedtime.

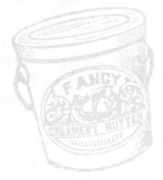

Onions by themselves—plain or cooked—have a long history of alleged curative powers. Biting into a large strong-tasting raw onion is sometimes advised for head colds; it will clean out the sinus passages but will probably kill your taste buds and surely destroy your desire for onions in any shape or form for some time to come. Onion soup made from a flavorful homemade beef stock is a better remedy, if only because it's more pleasant—certainly more palatable. The claims for onion soup stretch from a cold remedy to a bronchial treatment to a sure turnaround for the lovelorn.

ONION COUGH CURE

Makes 1 serving

1 large onion, sliced in thin rounds
½ cup lemon juice
1 cup sugar
Dash of cinnamon

Preheat the oven to 300°F.

Place the onion slices in an ovenproof bowl. Sprinkle the lemon juice over the slices, then add the sugar and cinnamon. Place the dish in the oven and bake for about 2 hours, or until the sugar is melted and the onion slices are soft.

Pour the juice that has collected in the bottom of the bowl into a cup and discard the onion. Sip the juice warm as required for sore throats or cough.

SYRUP OF TURNIP

Makes about four 1-teaspoon doses

The heavy sweet syrup, with a lingering taste of earthiness, calms a cough as it slips down your throat. This may sound downright awful; however, turnips are especially rich in vitamin C, just what your body needs to combat those nasty germs.

3 small young turnips
About ½ cup brown
    sugar

Pare and slice the turnips crosswise. Lay half the turnip slices on a wire rack placed over a bowl. Sprinkle half the brown sugar over the slices. Layer the rest of the slices over top and sprinkle them with the rest of the sugar. (Add more brown sugar if you need to.)

Place on top a plate that fits neatly over the turnips and weight it down. Let stand a few hours. Remove the plate, discard the turnips (or dot with butter and cook them in the oven—350°F for about 30 minutes—to use for the evening's meal), and drink the syrup that has collected in the bowl.

. . .

My FAVORITE over-the-counter cough medicine was given to me by my children's pediatrician, who confided that she was first introduced to it by her own children's Scottish nanny. It is based on Drambuie. Certainly a lot more expensive than Robitussin, but infinitely easier to swallow, this little cure is great for the last straggling ends of a cold and cough, when you're just so tired of being sick.

My pediatrician, who in all the years I knew her never once showed a glimmer of understatement, added, "It seems to cure the last of a sore throat and, if you take enough, it is certain to help you sleep." And indeed it does.

DRAMBUIE COUGH CURE

Makes about six 1-tablespoon doses

2 tablespoons Drambuie

¼ cup honey

Place the ingredients in a small jar with a tight lid. Close the lid and shake well. Take a spoonful as often as you wish.

Plumbing's All Messed Up

Indigestion, Nausea, Diarrhea, Constipation

One of the many comforts to be found in remedy recipes is the confidence with which they are written. Whether recorded by eminent physicians of the day or jotted down in household accounts and family cookbooks, these recipes are related in a reassuring manner, with phrases such as "this will cure for sure," or "in my experience this has always proven beneficial," tacked on to them. Tried out and perfected over the years, the recipes read like the gospel; half of their power seemed to reside in the strong faith that people placed in them.

Descriptions of recipes for healing the lower digestive tract are even more emphatic about their effectiveness than those for most other problem areas. Perhaps this is because nothing causes so much distress or dread than their particular symptoms. Nausea and indigestion can make grown men curl up like babies. Diarrhea and constipation will prevent the busiest woman from completing her chores. I've known people to work through severe colds, fevers, and even labor pains, while stomach rumblings and other gnawings around that area reduce them to a whimpering mess.

So we truly want to believe in a cure—anything that will ease the discomfort. Fortunately, these age-old recipes tend to have a sound basis in good medical sense. Here are the directions given in 1901 by Dr. Alcinous B. Jamison in his book, aptly named *Intestinal Ills*, to combat any kind of stomach pain: "The food should be nutritious and nonirritating. Reliance must be placed on liquid foods and beverages; in more acute cases it is well to stop all food for twelve or twenty-four hours." Jamison then goes on to recommend, first and foremost, pure spring water, toast, or rice water, four-day-old kefir (fermented milk), lactic-acid water, and milk diluted by a third with limewater. Acceptable food choices include chicken, mutton, or clam soups; minced chicken, filet of beef, sweetbreads; raw oysters; grapes without seeds or skins; rice boiled with milk; milk toast; mashed potatoes; and bread pudding. Foods to avoid are pork, veal, salt meats; fried or sugary foods; green leafy vegetables; and soups other than those mentioned.

All of this makes a great deal of sense, especially the suggestion to forgo food as soon as there is any hint of intestinal distress. But it is a curious aspect of human nature that we often *think* we want to eat precisely when we shouldn't.

In almost all but the most serious cases, stomach and intestinal problems are due to something impeding the natural flow of food through the body. The language that plumbers use to explain the workings of pipes is especially apt for this region of the body, which resembles nothing so much as a series of connecting tubes and a receptacle. Dr. F. Humphreys, famous for his still available Humphreys' homeopathic medicines, in his book *Humphreys' Mentor* (1891), called the stomach "the body's sink in which all is washed and disposed of." When our plumbing is in good working order, it does a very efficient job of separating what the body needs from the superfluous and sending them both on their way—one to nourish and fuel the body, the other flushed out of the system as waste. When they're not working, however, our pipes will come to a grinding halt, occasionally causing us to emit the whining noise of a broken pipe.

If you are a generally healthy person, the directions for relief from all the resulting troubles—indigestion, nausea, diarrhea, and constipation—are very similar. Stop eating for at least the first day, two for serious bouts. Drink only water, not cold but slightly warm, either plain or in weak teas and other lightly flavored beverages. The rationale behind this is to help the body concentrate on what it has to do—rid itself of the irritant.

When the symptoms begin to subside, slowly add something more substantial with small servings of gruels and porridge, clear soups, well-chewed fish and meat. For at least a week (and often it would be of benefit to continue two or three weeks after all symptoms are gone), common sense should dictate that nothing should be eaten that would annoy the afflicted region: Avoid most spices, hard liquor, rich desserts, and hard-to-digest vegetables and fruits such as tomatoes, cabbage, and turnips.

Good judgment and astute observation are more important with intestinal ills than with any other malady because, while the more alarming outward symptoms of diarrhea and nausea may pass, the internal effects of the illness—particularly dehydration—may still be occurring. Regular hours for meals should be maintained and the serving sizes kept very small, to be increased only if the patient has shown no signs of distress for at least twenty-four hours. If symptoms continue beyond forty-eight hours, a doctor should be consulted immediately.

The recipes listed below are grouped to follow the course of the illness, beginning with clear liquids and progressing to solid food and strengtheners. Those most effective for specific ills are identified in the headnotes that accompany each recipe.

First Day of Stomach Upset: Liquids

TOAST WATER

Makes 1 serving

Toast water is a good settler for upset or weak stomachs. I make it for the early stages of any intestinal virus when nothing seems to sit well. This version comes from Fannie Farmer's *Food and Cookery for the Sick and Convalescent*. She recommends toasting stale bread which she claims is easier to digest. It can be served hot or cold, but I've found that the bread gets unpleasantly mushy when it's too cold, so I prepare it warm.

2   slices of stale
    bread
    Milk and sugar,
    optional

Cut off the crusts of the bread and toast the slices until golden brown.

Place one slice in a small mixing bowl and pour 1 cup of boiling water over it. Set aside to cool slightly. Strain into a teacup.

Cut the remaining toast slice into small cubes and sprinkle over the warm water in the teacup. Add a little milk and sugar to the patient's taste, if desired. This should be sipped gradually.

BARLEY WATER

Makes 1 quart, enough for 1 day's serving for 1 person

Barley water is very good for cleansing the kidneys. I have two versions of this recipe—one very plain and one with more flavor added. The plain one, consisting of just barley, salt, and water, comes with the directive: "The nastier the taste, the better the cure," which is certainly an apt description. The flavorful one, given here, is much more palatable. It comes from *The Rumford Complete Cook Book* by Lily Haxworth Wallace ("Lecturer, Teacher and Writer on Domestic Science" is noted under her name on the flyleaf).

2 tablespoons pearl barley

⅓ teaspoon salt

Juice of ½ lemon

Sugar

Rinse the barley in a fine sieve, then place it in the top of a double boiler. Add 1 quart cold water and let the barley soak for 2 to 3 hours until soft. Add the salt and place the top of the double boiler over simmering water. Cook for at least 3 hours, stirring occasionally.

Strain the water through cheesecloth or a fine sieve into a glass pitcher. Flavor with lemon juice and add sugar to taste. Refrigerate until needed. Bring to room temperature or heat slightly when ready to serve.

APPLE WATER

Makes about 1 quart

A refreshing drink, very good for constipation. It does not keep very long—two days at the most—but it is very effective. Apple water can be served cold or slightly heated, with the addition of small pieces of dry toast.

1   pound flavorful apples such as golden russets, Macouns, Granny Smiths, winesaps, or Idareds

2¼ cups packed brown sugar

Preheat the oven to 350°F.

Cut the apples into quarters and bake them in a baking pan until the flesh is easily pricked with a fork. Put them immediately into a very large container, preferably glass or ceramic, and cover with the brown sugar.

Pour 1 gallon boiling water over the apples. Let stand until the water cools. Drain the apples and press them through a fine sieve or process them in batches in a food processor fitted with the metal blade. Strain through cheesecloth or a fine sieve into a bowl, and discard the pulp.

APPLE SOUP

Makes four ½-cup servings

Chef Alexis Soyer recommended apple soup not only for constipation but as an autumn tonic, useful for cleansing the body of summer's excesses. I have also served the soup as a first course at a dinner party, coupled with a pork roast as the main dish for the first bracing night of November.

3 pounds baking apples, peeled, cored, and quartered

2 teaspoons cornstarch

1½ tablespoons sugar

1 teaspoon cinnamon

Salt

In a large saucepan, stew the apples in 2 cups of water until very soft. In a small bowl, mix the cornstarch, sugar, and cinnamon with 2 teaspoons water to form a smooth paste. Pour into the apples, bring to a boil, and simmer for 5 minutes. Add salt to taste.

Serve with dry or very lightly buttered toast points.

BERRY GELATIN

Makes 1 serving

You can use either strawberries or raspberries for this recipe. Both are good for queasy stomachs. The Amish, from whom this recipe comes, also recommend gelatin drinks for the elderly who cannot sleep at night.

1   packet unflavored gelatin

1   cup fresh strawberries or raspberries

Dissolve the gelatin in 1 cup boiling water. Press the berries through a fine sieve. Discard the seeds and add the pulp to the gelatin water. Serve hot or slightly warm.

◦§   WATERMELON   §◦

Normally, one should drink at least eight glasses of water daily, but more should be consumed with any digestive track ailments, especially diarrhea. Eating a whole or a great part of a watermelon was often advised if this amount of water was hard to get down. Melon is a terrific way to replenish fluids and it will help soothe stomach cramps.

· · ·

JOHN MILNER FOTHERGILL was a member of the London Society of Physicians when he wrote *Food for the Invalid; The Convalescent; The Dyspeptic; and The Gouty* in 1880. He comes across in his book as a very compassionate man who doesn't like to be second-guessed. ("The attending physician should never question the members of the household [about the patient] as it may cloud his judgement," he states in his preface.) The recipes he records in his book are fairly common but some of them betray his patrician class in the rarity of ingredients and skill needed in their preparation. These dishes—more suited for banquets than the sickroom—would make a rich person comfortable during recovery.

MILK AND BRANDY

Makes 1 serving

Milk and brandy, however, was a common—and favorite—beverage among all classes when dealing with a sour stomach. It is especially comforting before an afternoon nap or at bedtime.

1 cup milk	Warm the milk gently in a small saucepan.
1 teaspoon good quality brandy	Pour into a glass and stir in the brandy and powdered sugar. Dust with nutmeg to taste
1 teaspoon confectioners' sugar	and serve immediately.
Nutmeg	

WHITE WINE WHEY

Makes 1 serving

The note accompanying this recipe in *Madam Johnson's Presents (or Every Young Woman's Companion in Useful and Universal Knowledge)* by Madam Johnson (1770), an English noblewoman with an estate in Ireland, says it is a helpful drink for cramping and stomach weaknesses, as well as for "feminine nervous complaints."

1   cup hot milk

1 or 2 wineglasses full of good-quality white wine (depending, I guess, on severity of distress or nerves)

Powdered sugar

Add the wine to the milk and stir in powdered sugar to taste. Sip slowly, lying down.

Teas

Certain kinds of herbal teas are very good for indigestion and nausea. The important thing to remember is to sip the teas slowly—a very little bit at a steady pace. The steady rhythm may also help recovery, as it slows down the body.

GINGER TEA

Makes 1 serving

Ginger is a powerful stimulant to the digestive organs and is particularly good for nausea, seasickness, menstrual cramps, sour stomach, gas or bloating, and is especially useful after any abdominal surgery.

1 cup weak tea (such as Earl Grey, Irish Breakfast, or Chinese green leaf, but avoid using another herbal tea)

1-inch piece of fresh ginger, peeled

Sugar or honey

Prepare the tea in your usual way. Bruise the ginger by crushing it gently with the flat side of a broad knife (this releases the juices).

Place the ginger in the tea and let steep for 5 minutes. For severe cases you can leave the ginger in the tea, where it will continue to release its juices, but it can also be removed. Add sweetener to taste. Sip slowly.

RASPBERRY LEAF TEA

Makes about 3 servings

Raspberry leaves have been relied upon for hundreds of years to counteract diarrhea. Begin to sip this tea after the first bout and drink several small cups throughout the day.

2 teaspoons finely crumbled dried raspberry leaves

Sugar

Place the crumbled leaves in a tea strainer. Bring 2 cups water to a boil. Let the leaves steep in the water for at least 5 minutes.

Drink hot or cold, sweetened with a little sugar.

PEPPERMINT TEA

Makes 1 serving

This is good for nausea. You can buy peppermint tea bags in a health food store, but the following recipe is more pleasing—and a little faster-acting.

4 or 5 large peppermint leaves, washed and cut into fine strips

2 cloves, lightly crushed

1 cinnamon stick

Place peppermint leaf strips in a tea infuser or a small sieve and pour about 1 cup boiling water over them into a teacup. Let steep a few minutes.

Stir the crushed cloves into the tea. Stir with the cinnamon stick.

CHAMOMILE TEA

Makes about 4 servings

Chamomile was suggested for two reasons by Dr. Robert Wallace Johnson: It strengthens the stomach, especially after bouts of vomiting, and it calms the nerves. To follow the directions given, gather blossoms in July when many parks and roadsides are blooming with the fragrant herb. You may also substitute for the blossoms the prepared tea bags found in most stores, but the tea won't be nearly as effective. Just make sure the store-bought tea is the freshest available; the longer it has been on the shelf, the less potent it becomes.

½ tablespoon chamomile blossoms

Place the blossoms in a stainless steel saucepan and add 1 pint water. Bring to a boil, then quickly remove from heat. Cover and let stand for half an hour. Strain before serving.

AGRIMONY

Makes 1 serving

Agrimony is usually found in health food stores already packaged as teabags. A flowering herb common to England, it can sometimes be found fresh in fancy food stores. It is a very good diuretic, highly recommended to flush out toxins in the body.

If the agrimony is fresh, use about 1 tablespoon of the stem, leaves, and flowers. Pour about 1 cup hot water over the agrimony into a teacup and let steep a few minutes. Do not add sweeteners.

. . .

THE VAN RENSSELAERS were a very prosperous landowning family in New York. In 1835, the female head, Maria, published a selection of recipes. The family's recipes show them to have been a funny bunch (intentionally or not, I don't know), with decided preferences and prejudices. I talk more about them in the chapter on tonics and first aid remedies. But the one thing that must be said here is that they were patriots who fought the British well (they were, after all, Dutch patricians). Among their numbers were a few doctors, and the following recipe comes from them. The headnote attached to it reads, "For a bloody flux, it cured our Soldiers in our war."

SWEET FERN TEA

Makes about 4 servings

½ cup fiddlehead ferns (available at farmers markets)

Place the ferns in a teapot and add 2 cups boiling water. Let steep at least 5 minutes. Serve without benefit of sweeteners.

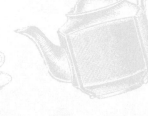

BEEF TEA

Makes about 2 servings

Freshly made beef tea used to be the mainstay of an invalid's daily menu. Essentially, it is comprised of the juices from a raw round steak, and it was thought to contain a lot of much-needed protein. However, Miss Nightingale stated in *Notes on Nursing* that many patients were actually starving to death because their care-givers were relying too heavily on the supposed nutritional benefits of beef teas.

In fact, beef tea is nothing more than a sort of homemade bouillon, rather salty, but easy on the stomach. It is equally useful for queasy stomachs and stuffy colds when a hot liquid will open up the chest a bit. This version is from *The Rumford Complete Cook Book*.

½ pound top of round steak

½ pint cold water

⅓ level teaspoon kosher salt

Cut the meat in small pieces (the smaller the pieces, the more easily it will give off its juices, or you may scrape the meat from the fiber). Place the meat in a medium-size bowl and add the cold water. Let stand for half an hour.

Pour the meat and the liquid into a medium-size sauce pan and slowly bring to a slow simmer. Let it simmer for 1 hour. (Add more water if needed.) Strain and season with salt.

Beef tea may be served hot or frozen, in which case it should be chopped up fine in a blender or a food processor. Can be stored for 1 day.

CURE FOR THE PILES

Makes enough for about 1 week

You don't get much blunter than this. Another recipe which works well for constipation, from the Van Rensselaers' treasure trove, dated July 23, 1830.

2 quarts flat beer	Mix beer, prunes, and currants together in a large stainless steel saucepan. Bring to a boil and reduce to one-half the original quantity. Remove from the heat, pour into a container, and stir in the cassis. Cover and refrigerate. Keeps for a week.
½ pound prunes	
¼ pound currants	
¼ cup cassis liqueur	

Take a teacup full of the juice once in the morning and once in the evening until relief comes.

TEETHING BABY RELIEF

My children are beyond the teething stage—praise the Lord—so to test this recipe out I coerced my brother to lend me his daughter, a bubbling, joyous bundle. It was a test of love for him—and his wife—as I described the recipe from Dr. William Hall, because they are both firm believers in children being nurtured only on naturally healthful food (except that Joe has been known to sneak his children gummy bears, and both my sister and I have corrupted them further with things like Raisinets and Tootsie Rolls, but we all take pains to hide these things from my sister-in-law). So here I was, advocating that their darling be allowed to chew on pork rind to combat the diarrhea associated with severe teething. They quickly shut up after it worked. The recipe is given as Dr. Hall wrote it in his text, *Health by Good Living* (1870).

> "For teething babies suffering from diarrhea; chew bacon rind with some fat attached. It seems to have a beneficial effect on the gums, also."

Second Day: Semiliquids and Soft Food

BEEF BROTH

Makes 1 serving

The addition of an egg yolk gives this broth an extra bit of nutrition.
It is very easy on the stomach.

½ pound round steak
or shin of beef
(which will yield
more gelatin)

1 large egg yolk

Salt

Cut the beef into small cubes, reserving the bone
if using shin. Place the meat in a medium bowl
and add 2 cups water. Let stand for half an hour.

Pour the meat and water into the top of
a double boiler set over simmering water. Add
the shin bone if using. Cook for 2 hours.
Strain and press as much of the meat pulp as
possible through the sieve. Discard the solids.
Keep the broth warm.

Lightly beat the egg yolk and 2 tablespoons
of the broth in a small saucepan. Cook over
medium heat, stirring constantly, until the
mixture coats a spoon with a thin film, or has
reached 160°F.

Place the yolk mixture in a warm bowl.
Add the warm broth and season lightly with
salt. Serve immediately.

CHICKEN SOUP FOR THE CHALLENGED STOMACH

Makes about 6 servings

The difference between this chicken soup and the one given in the chapter on colds and flus is that this is very plain and *all* fat has been carefully removed to make it as gentle as possible on the stomach. Add rice to combat diarrhea.

1 boiling fowl
1 tablespoon salt
½ cup cooked rice, optional

Place the fowl in a large stockpot and cover with 3 quarts water. Add the salt and simmer gently for 4 hours.

Remove the fowl from the broth, pick off the chicken that remains on the bones, and reserve in a separate bowl. With a slotted spoon, remove the meat that has fallen into the broth. Strain the broth through cheesecloth or a fine sieve several times. Store the broth in a container and refrigerate. Refrigerate the chicken separately.

When the broth is cold, skim off all the fat on the top.

To serve, heat only as much broth as you require at a time. Season with a little salt. If you wish to add rice, stir in about a tablespoon of cooked rice just before serving.

CHICKEN JELLY

Makes 2 servings

The chicken from the previous recipe is so light on the stomach and so nutritious, it simply should not be wasted. The recipe was found in Marion Harland's *Common Sense in the Household* (1871).

2 cups boiled chicken meat

Salt and pepper

1 tablespoon unflavored gelatin

½ cup chicken broth

Pound the meat until it resembles "white rags." Press through a sieve into a bowl and season with salt and pepper to taste. In a medium bowl sprinkle the gelatin over the broth and let stand until it softens. Stir in the chicken meat until well mixed. Place mixture in a mold and refrigerate until firm. Serve cold, either plain or on good bread or plain crackers.

OATMEAL GRUEL

Makes 1 serving

Fannie Farmer swore that oatmeal gruel was good for nursing mothers. She claimed it made their milk more plentiful and added to their strength as well. I have also found this very good to counteract diarrhea, if given in small servings.

1 cup milk or water (or half of each)

¼ teaspoon kosher salt

2 tablespoons Irish oatmeal (rolled oats will do but Irish oatmeal is more flavorful)

Pinch of cinnamon, optional

Fruit jelly, optional

Bring the water or milk (or a combination) and salt to a boil over direct heat in the top of a double boiler and stir in the oats. Cook for 15 minutes.

Place the pan over the bottom of the boiler and cook over gently simmering water for 1 hour.

Strain the gruel through cheesecloth for a smoother consistency or leave as is. If you like, add a pinch of cinnamon or a little fruit jelly to flavor.

FLAVORFUL GRUEL

Makes 1 serving

This recipe on the microfilm copy of Dr. Robert Wallace Johnson's book, *Nurse's Guide and Family Assistance,* bore the original handwritten tracing, "Papa's favorite!" Seeing the faded ink made me realize how much these recipes had been relied upon and used.

Unlike the other recipes using fairly raw eggs, I do not direct you to cook the egg any more than it will cook in the oatmeal. In my testing, the egg was sufficiently cooked when the farina or cream of wheat was poured over it. Just make sure the gruel is steaming hot. If you're still uneasy about any escaping bacteria, follow the directions for using raw eggs on pages 13–14.

1 cup prepared farina or cream of wheat

1 thin strip of lemon zest

1 large egg, beaten to a froth

1 wineglass of sherry (about ½ cup)

1 teaspoon sugar

Nutmeg

Prepare the farina or cream of wheat according to the directions on the box, adding the lemon zest while it cooks. When the cereal is done, discard the peel.

Pour the very hot farina or cream of wheat into a serving bowl. Stir in the egg, wine, sugar, and nutmeg to taste.

For extra bulk, especially when recovering from diarrhea or nausea, you can serve this with snippets of dry toast stirred into it.

SAPS (MILK TOAST)

Makes 1 serving

When I was growing up I never tasted milk toast, but I did hear jokes about it—or rather, heard the name used to describe someone who was weak. After tasting milk toast, however, I think it's a wonderful description for comfort and security. It's a perfect dish for the day after a serious bout of nausea or diarrhea. It settles the stomach in a warm way, adding just the right amount of weight.

1 slice flavorful white bread

1 tablespoon sugar

½ cup cream or milk, slightly warmed

Break the bread into a cup and pour ½ cup boiling water over it. Place a saucer on top of the cup to retain the steam for a minute or two. Drain off the excess water and stir in the sugar. Mix with a spoon. Add the cream or milk (use cream only if the patient is not experiencing diarrhea) and serve at once.

STEWED PLUMS

Makes about 6 servings

Sometimes after a bout of diarrhea, constipation sets in. This recipe from the wonderful Alexis Soyer will relieve the symptoms.

12 medium Italian or prune plums, peeled and pitted

1 teaspoon brown sugar

Pinch of cinnamon

Zest of 1 lemon

Small wineglass (about ¼ cup) port or sherry

Place the plums in a large saucepan and add just enough water to cover them. Let sit for half an hour, then add the brown sugar, ½ cup water, the cinnamon, and lemon zest. Bring to a gentle simmer and let stew for 20 minutes.

Transfer the plums to a bowl and refrigerate until chilled. Just before serving, stir in the wine. The syrup from the plums is beneficial by itself.

APPLESAUCE

Makes about 4 servings

My mom would make this for us when we were constipated, or for what she called "the willies," which was her term for nothing being truly wrong with us except that we were grumpy. It helped.

1 pound cooking apples

1 cup sugar

1 tablespoon cinnamon

Peel, core, and quarter the apples. Place them in a pan with the sugar and ⅓ cup water. Bring to a boil and simmer until soft, about 20 minutes.

Remove from heat and pour almost all the water from the apples. With a fork or potato ricer, mash the apples to a chunky pulp. Sprinkle with cinnamon. Serve warm (delicious and gratifying) or at room temperature.

HASTY PUDDING FOR CHILDREN'S BREAKFAST

Makes 1 serving

The very model of a nursery dish! When anyone under my roof has a tummyache, this is what they get. For serious cases, serve it plain. For those times when a stomachache is caused by the blues or a hostile world, stir in a teaspoon of your best jam (for adults, float a good puddle of your best liquor on top, as well). Then wrap the sufferer in your fluffiest quilt or softest blanket and sit close to him on a bed mounded with pillows with your arms protectively surrounding him.

1 cup plus 2 teaspoons fresh milk

2 teaspoons flour

Jam or cinnamon, optional

Bring the 1 cup of milk to a boil in a small saucepan. Remove from heat.

In a small bowl, mix the flour with the remaining 2 teaspoons milk and add to the hot milk. Stir until the milk thickens.

Serve plain, or with a flavoring such as jam or cinnamon if you prefer.

Third Day and General Convalescence: Gradual Return to Normal Diet

CORNMEAL BREAKFAST CAKE

Makes 4 servings

Margaret J. Thompson's book *Food for the Sick and Well* (1920) is filled with very strict rules for dealing with intestinal disorders. Mrs. Thompson believed that for as long as a week the patient should be given no food. At the end of that time the patient would be allowed something hefty like this dish. I think she's rather overcautious, but some cases may warrant such treatment. In any case, these cakes are a delicious greeting for the truly starved convalescent.

2 cups cornmeal

2 tablespoons wheat flour

1 tablespoon sugar

1 teaspoon salt

1 teaspoon baking soda

2 teaspoons cream of tartar

Preheat the oven to 350°F.

Mix together the cornmeal and flour in a medium bowl. Add the sugar, salt, baking soda, and cream of tartar and stir well.

Mix together the milk, egg, and butter in a small bowl. Make a well in the center of the cornmeal mixture and add the liquid all at once. Stir quickly to mix well.

2 cups milk

1 large egg, beaten

3 tablespoons melted butter

Bake in a well-greased shallow 1-quart baking dish for 20 minutes, until the cake puffs up golden and the center is firm to the touch. You can also test by inserting a skewer in the center, if it comes out clean, it's done.

Serve with a little melted butter or good maple syrup.

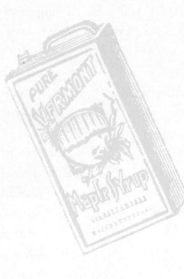

DAINTY PUDDING

Makes 1 serving

The recipe for this pudding was given to me by an elderly cousin of my mother-in-law. She said that she was served this when she was child whenever she was constipated—or whenever her nurse thought she was constipated: "If I was in a temper or out of sorts in some way, out came dainty pudding!"

Two thin slices of stale white bread, crusts removed

½ cup hot, fresh, peeled and pitted stewed plums

Warm cream

Cut the bread into pieces about 3 inches long and 1 inch wide. Line a small bowl with the bread pieces, fitting them closely together. Spread the hot fruit over the bread, then place more bread on top.

Fit a saucer inside the bowl right on top of the bread. Weigh the plate down and set aside until the fruit cools, about 30 minutes.

Remove the saucer and turn the pudding out on a plate. Serve with a little custard sauce or warm cream.

SAVORY CUSTARD

Makes 2 servings

This is a good way to begin reintroducing solid food to someone who has been experiencing bouts of nausea or indigestion.

2 large eggs
   Salt and pepper
1 cup hot Beef Tea
   (page 87)

Beat the eggs until light but not foamy in a medium mixing bowl. Add salt and pepper to taste. Pour the hot beef tea over the eggs. Strain the mixture into slightly greased custard cups.

To cook the custard on the stove, place the cups in a wide saucepan and pour hot water into the pan to come about two-thirds of the way up the cups. Cover the pan and simmer gently (adding more hot water as necessary) until a knife blade inserted in the custard comes out clean, about 30 minutes.

To bake the custards, preheat the oven to 275°F. Place the custard cups in an ovenproof dish and pour hot water into the dish to come about two-thirds of the way up the cups. Bake for about 25 minutes, or until a knife blade inserted in the custard comes out clean.

CUSTARD SOUFFLÉ

Makes 2 servings

As light as air, this custard is good to nourish a weak and empty stomach. It is fairly easy to digest and will make the patient feel satisfyingly full.

2 teaspoons butter, plus a bit for greasing the cups

1 tablespoon flour

⅓ cup milk

1 large egg, separated

1 tablespoon sugar

Preheat the oven to 350°F. Grease 2 custard cups with butter and set aside.

Melt the butter in a medium saucepan and add the flour. Stir to blend well but do not let brown. Pour in the milk and stir until the flour is dissolved. Allow the milk to come to a gentle boil and cook for 3 minutes more, stirring constantly. Remove from heat.

Beat the egg yolk to a light lemon color in a medium bowl. In a separate bowl, with clean beaters, whip the egg white until stiff peaks form. Pour the hot milk into the yolk and stir to mix. Add the sugar and stir. Gently fold in the egg white.

Turn the mixture into the prepared custard cups and bake in the center of the oven until firm, about 15 minutes. Serve at once.

CURDS AND WHEY

Makes 1 serving

I had to look up rennet for this recipe; finding it was another story. For those who are as ignorant as I am, rennet is extracted (in a most horrible-sounding process) from the membrane lining the fourth stomach of a cow. It was used to curdle milk for cheese and puddings. Fortunately, rennet is now available in powdered or tablet form in most well-stocked gourmet or health food stores. I've also seen it listed in a specialty baking catalog.

The recipe I have uses the term *blood heat* to describe how hot you want the milk to be. I love the term but have changed it for more clarity. Besides bringing up nursery images, curds and whey is a very good dish for someone requiring a light diet, especially useful after a bout of nausea and indigestion.

2 cups milk	Bring the milk to the point just before it
1½ teaspoons rennet powder	begins to boil in a small saucepan. Remove from the heat and add the rennet. Stir well.
½ teaspoon vanilla extract	Add vanilla and pour into a pretty serving dish. Let cool to room temperature.
Fruit jam, optional	If more sweetness is desired, stir in a teaspoon or two of fruit jam.

SNOW PUDDING

Makes four ½-cup servings

Dr. Fothergill related that his cook made a very good snow pudding. He doesn't give her name, but her pudding is a fine memorial. It is recommended both for indigestion and for general convalescence.

1 package unflavored gelatin

1 cup sugar

Juice of 2 large lemons

2 large egg whites

⅛ teaspoon cream of tartar

Mix I cup cold water with the gelatin in a medium bowl. Let the gelatin soften, then add 2 cups boiling water, the sugar, and the lemon juice. Stir until well mixed. Strain through a fine sieve to remove any lemon pulp and let stand, refrigerated, until just set, about I hour.

Place the egg whites, 2 tablespoons water, and the cream of tartar in a heavy saucepan. Cook over very low heat, beating constantly with a wire whisk, to a temperature of 160°F. Pour into a medium bowl and beat the whites until stiff. Fold gently into the chilled gelatin mixture. Pour into a mold and refrigerate until set, about 4 hours.

TAPIOCA JELLY

Makes 2 servings

Hardly anyone I know seems to like tapioca because they've never tasted the real thing. This recipe, however, has changed minds. It will help indigestion and has been known to ease the restless into a good night's sleep.

⅓ cup tapioca

⅓ cup sugar

Juice and grated zest of 1 lemon

2 tablespoons sherry or 1 tablespoon of brandy

In the top of a double boiler set on direct heat, bring 1½ cups water to a boil and add the tapioca. Stir to mix well. Let cook until slightly thickened; then remove from heat. You can strain it through a fine sieve if you want a smooth jelly, or leave it as is.

Add the sugar and lemon juice and zest and stir well. Let cool, then add the wine or brandy. Pour into 2 serving cups and refrigerate to set.

PUFFED EGG

Makes 1 serving

Try this to settle a slightly queasy stomach.

1 large egg,
separated

Pinch of salt

Pepper

Beat the egg white until stiff. Add the salt. Turn the white into a custard cup and place in a saucepan. Pour into the saucepan enough warm water to come two-thirds of the way up the custard cup.

Cover the saucepan with a lid and steam the custard for 3 minutes. Remove the lid. If the white has puffed up, drop the unbroken yolk into the center of the white (if it hasn't puffed up, put the lid back on and steam another minute or two, then add the yolk). Replace the lid and cook until the yolk is just set.

Carefully remove the custard cup from the hot water with tongs, place on a saucer, and serve warm with a little salt and pepper.

PRAWN SOUP

Makes about 6 servings

This is one of the fancy recipes from Dr. Fothergill. He recommends the soup for indigestion, convalescence, and gout. It is a beautiful soup no matter how you feel, but it is very nice to serve to patients who are just recovering and beginning to feel the first pangs of health return. It will make them feel very special, indeed. An added benefit is that the whole family will enjoy the soup at the same time.

1 very lively lobster (female if possible, to collect the roe sack)

2 tablespoons butter

1 medium onion, thinly sliced

2½ quarts fish stock or chicken stock, preferably homemade

¼ cup flour

50 prawns or small shrimp, shells and heads removed

Salt and pepper

Quickly kill the lobster by inserting a knife at the base of its head. Cut the meat from the lobster shell, including the claws, into small pieces. Scoop out as much of the roe sack as you can. Tear or cut the lobster shell into several pieces.

Melt the butter in a medium stockpot and sauté the onion until translucent. Add the lobster meat, roe, lobster shell, and claws. Stir once or twice, then add 1 quart of water. Bring to a gentle boil and cook for 1 hour. Remove from heat and strain the stock through a fine sieve into a large bowl. With the back of a large spoon, press all the liquid you can from the meat and shells. Pick the

shells out from among the roe and meat.
Discard the shells. Save the meat and roe for
another use (it does not go back into the
soup). Return the lobster stock to a clean pot
and add the fish or chicken stock. Bring to a
simmer.

In a small bowl, mix the flour with ½ cup
of the hot stock to make a paste. Stir the flour
paste into the rest of the stock and simmer
the stock, stirring occasionally, until it
thickens. Raise the heat higher and bring
the stock to a boil, then cook 30 minutes
longer. Strain the stock again.

Return the stock to a clean pot. Add
the prawns or shrimp and simmer until the
shellfish turns pink and is cooked through.
Season with salt and pepper to taste.

BEEF CAKES

Makes 1 serving

The Rumford Complete Cook Book notes that beef cakes are a very good way to reintroduce beef into the diet after an illness. What you have here is a hamburger made of very lean beef, but instead of the meat being ground it's scraped so it becomes almost shredded. I have recorded the recipe exactly as it is in the book because I like what it says about cooking for the sick.

¼ pound very lean round steak

Salt and pepper

Toast

Cut the meat into strips, remove every particle of fat, and scrape the pulp from the fiber of the meat. Season lightly, remembering that the palate is more sensitive to seasonings in sickness than in health. Form into very small balls or cakes, and broil on both sides until well cooked. Serve on rounds of buttered or dry toast.

BOILED LAMB SWEETBREADS

Makes 4 servings

Sweetbreads have a reputation as a fortifier—they are a rich source of vitamins and proteins. This must be the reason why there are so many sweetbread recipes in invalid cooking. I have selected two—the lamb, which is very plain, and a veal, which has a little more flavor. Whether they're fortifiers or not, I have found sweetbreads to be a very light meal, especially good for indigestion and that rickety stage after nausea and diarrhea.

1 pound lamb sweetbreads

Salt

2 cups milk

3 tablespoons flour

Toast

Clean the sweetbreads and sprinkle them with salt. Remove all the tissues, cover with water, and let stand a few hours with a little salt.

Drain and wash the sweetbreads again, then pat dry and place in a medium saucepan. Add the milk and simmer gently for about 45 minutes or until the sweetbreads are tender.

Remove the sweetbreads with a slotted spoon to a warm plate. Keep warm while you make the sauce. Add the flour to the milk, stirring until all the lumps are removed and the sauce thickens. Pour the sauce over the sweetbreads and serve at once with toast points.

SWEETBREADS À LA NEWBURG

Makes 2 servings

I would serve this dish a little later on in an illness, when the patient is all but recovered but maybe just a little depressed and in need of an elegant dining experience. Use the best sweetbreads you can find—what's called the "heart"—and serve them on your finest china.

1 pair veal sweetbreads

3 tablespoons unsalted butter

1 cup half-and-half

2 large egg yolks, well beaten

2 tablespoons sherry

Salt and pepper

4 slices of toast

Parboil the sweetbreads in a medium saucepan filled with lightly salted water until slightly tender, then cut them in cubes. Reserve.

Melt the butter in a large skillet. Add the cubes of sweetbread and sauté for 5 minutes. Add the cream and cook gently 5 minutes longer. Add the egg yolks, stirring constantly, and cook until the sauce thickens. Be careful not to let it boil. Add the sherry and salt and pepper to taste and stir to mix well.

Cut the toast into points and arrange on plates. Spoon the sweetbreads into the middle, then pour the sauce over them. Serve at once.

STEAMED LEMON SOLE

Makes 2 servings

Sole is a common dish for the convalescent because of its delicate taste. When cooking fish for someone just getting over an illness—particularly a stomach illness—always make the effort to go to a good fish store. The fish must always be very fresh; you don't want a strong smell in the house, or compromised taste.

Salt and pepper
4 sole fillets
1 lemon

Salt and pepper each fillet. Roll the fillets up and lay them in a steamer insert. Squeeze the lemon over the fillets.

Bring a medium saucepan of water to a boil. Set the steamer of fish over the boiling water and cover with a pot lid (a size slightly smaller than the steamer will do). Let steam for about 20 minutes, or until the fish is tender.

HADDOCK IN MILK

Makes 2 servings

My second cousin, Mary Dougherty, gave this recipe to my mother when she heard about my interest in cooking for the sick. She told my mom that when she married her husband, Hugh, his mother Margaret (my grandmother's sister) taught her how to cook this dish because Hugh had a delicate stomach. Hugh was the head of prison guards at a state penitentiary. He stood 6 feet 4 inches tall and was about as robust a man as you'd ever want to meet. From what I could observe at family parties, his delicate constitution was solely in his mother's eyes.

Nevertheless, this is a very nice dish and one of the few fish preparations I have found that my family will eat, delicate stomachs or not.

Four 4-ounce haddock fillets
Salt and pepper
1½ teaspoons herbes de Provence
2 cups milk
8 tablespoons (1 stick) butter
1 cup heavy cream
1½ tablespoons flour
Toast points

Season the fillets with salt and pepper to taste and the herbs. Arrange the fillets in a stainless steel or enamel skillet and add the milk. Bring the milk to a gentle simmer and cook the fish until it's tender and begins to flake, about 10 minutes.

Remove the fillets with a slotted spoon to a plate and keep warm while you make the sauce. Add the butter to the milk and melt, stirring occasionally. Add the cream and stir, then let the sauce come back to a simmer. Add the flour, stirring constantly to avoid lumping. Cook over low heat until the sauce thickens a little. (It will be a thin sauce, in any case.)

Arrange the toast points on 2 plates. Arrange 2 fillets per person over the toast points. Pour a little of the sauce over the fish and serve the remaining sauce on the side.

Not Feeling Yourself

Strengtheners, Restoratives, Amusements

The hardest thing to admit to yourself when you're taking care of anyone who is sick—from your beloved partner to your cherished child—is just how much work it is. Every waking hour is dedicated to the sufferer lying in bed. You think about what will make them more comfortable, what will relieve the ever-changing symptoms as the illness progresses from day to day. You long for their contentment; play endless card games, bring them books, new magazines, the newspaper still neatly folded (you don't have time to read it yourself). Mealtime becomes more troublesome. Even during those periods when eating is difficult, it remains a much anticipated focal point in the patient's long day while the care-giver's anxiety mounts over what can be served that will not hamper, and will hopefully speed, the longed-for recovery.

More than likely you're also working, or attempting to work. A few days are wriggled free at home from the boss, but then you have to return—and find yourself calling a couple of times a day to make sure the patient hasn't succumbed in your absence. At the end of the day, you rush home, cursing the subways, the traffic, the person before you in the supermarket line who insists on telling a funny story to the checkout lady when you are absolutely certain that, if you don't get to your charge in the next minute or two, it will all be over.

And what do you get for all this? Just the small miracles of your patient's revival, and life drifting back to its former shape. It is the patient who, still appearing wan, will gather sympathy from all who hear of the horrible passage past the jaws of death while you are rarely afforded much more than an acknowledging nod. You are, however, exhausted, utterly depleted. And, under a rattling lid of guilt, just a bit annoyed.

"It is your duty," Marion Harland chided a young woman in her popular handbook *Common Sense in the Household.* (Harland was the pen name for the proper housewife Mary Virginia Hawes Terhune who made a tidy mint with this and other books of advice on refined Christian living that she published throughout the late 1800s.) "I would not forget, or let you forget for a moment, the truth that the sick is the greater sufferer."

Mrs. Harland recorded this advice after hearing the woman complain about nursing her husband and three small children all at once through the flu. On top of this ghastly occurrence (in a period when even the most common flu strains were a great danger), one of her servants quit and the weather outside was so chilly and muddy that the house could not be kept either warm or clean.

"I am fairly wild!" Mrs. Harland reports the poor woman screaming at her. "I cannot snatch a minute, from morning until night, to put things straight, and yet I am almost tired to death! I was saying to myself as you came in that I wouldn't try any longer. I would just sit still until the dirt was piled up to my chin, and *then I would get upon the table!*"

I, for one, was happy to come across this passage and by no means for Mrs. Harland's advice, which I consider pretty cruel. A good long movie and a drink or two in a quiet bar afterward would have been my solution. Rather, I appreciate this woman's despairing anger. Her all-too-human surrender to a maddening situation is a rare admission in these documents, in which most women are portrayed as tending to the sickroom with nothing short of abiding fortitude and patience. When I wade through these narratives it is with the uneasy awareness that, by the third day of any nursing bout, I am usually tempted to snap at my charges to get up and get their own damn glass of juice. In calm, rational moments, I am apt to reason that, without modern hospitals or effective hygiene and medicine, such noble deportment was the conditional response to the frequency of serious illness that visited most households until the early twentieth century. There *was* nothing else to do but soldier on. But I also believe these accounts were often colored by Victorian society's widely held belief that women were constitutionally incapable of being anything less (or more) than compassionate angels. Even Miss Nightingale proclaimed, "Women are set by nature to be better nurses, for their quiet minds enable them to observe and to patiently wait upon the special requirements of the sick room." However, not all women were created equal in Nightingale's eyes. In *Notes on Nursing*, she ranks at the top of the competence ladder English women (of course)—superior in perception to French or Irish women, whom she deemed too quick to be sound observers, or German women, whom she considered too slow-witted.

Deep down inside, though, I've always had the nagging suspicion that, even then, the reality was far different. For while it is one of the nicest, most loving acts you can perform for another person—to get them through this time of suffering in the most comfortable (and humorous) manner possible—it is also hard and exhausting work. To do it right—all the tending, the observing, the delicate feeding that is required to return the body to health—all other concerns must be set aside, the care-giver's own life suppressed. In this demanding climate, even the most diligent, self-sacrificing person—man or woman—must surely begin to feel depleted after awhile. Not to acknowledge this is, to my mind, oppressively heartless, and while it's right that the emphasis should remain on the patient, some concern should also be extended to the weary nurse, as well.

And, yet, how rarely this occurs. In most incidents, the bloom of health peeking through the patient's cheeks is probably the only reward that is received. Once the work is done, most care-givers must make do with merely being allowed to take themselves off to their own beds for a well-earned and vital rest.

SOMETIMES, when I am sitting by myself in the twilight of a day spent with a sick child or friend, I find myself mulling over my guilt for not being a more compassionate and patient nurse. I'm convinced that much of the way you go through caring for the sick ultimately depends on the examples you grew up with and, most assuredly, on the bare reality of who you are—not on the face you put forward to the world, but on the genuine nature of your mettle. This may seem to be a very self-evident statement, but it is often conveniently overlooked.

For my part, I know it has taken me many years to comfortably acknowledge the fact that, as the days go by and my eyes cast increasingly colder glances on my charge, I am simply being unmasked as my mother's true daughter. She gave our family exactly twenty-four hours to get well before she'd stand beside our beds and, with hands on hips, cry, "Buck up and stop your belly-aching." Never admitting to feeling ill herself, she rarely missed a day of work, forging on through the same colds and flu that brought the rest of her family to an exasperated halt. She had no patience for weakness, which was, perhaps, a result of being just a little bit afraid of the neediness she saw in our eyes. Not one to gather her children in her arms (her formidable Irish disposition was convinced that we'd turn soft and spoil if she did), the best my mother could give us if she realized we were truly sick was to send our father into us. Aside from his more gentle and humorous disposition, he had been trained as a medical technician in England during World War II. He expertly pressed cooling towels to our feverish foreheads, made sure a pitcher of iced water was on the bedside table, and plumped the pillows at our backs while telling us stories to make us laugh.

I have spent a great deal of time freely wrapping my arms around my children. I bring jars of broth to friends and have sat long hours at the bedsides of ailing parents and relatives because of the care my father instilled in me. But, to be honest, most times I am struggling to quash the impatient disposition I inherited from my mother. Friends generally think of me as good-natured. I go through the day with what they consider to be a sort of calming grace, but few ever suspect the irritable heartlessness warring inside. Get up, get out, we have to get on with life, I want to shout at whomever I'm tending, pulling the sheets a little too roughly, making do with scrambled eggs instead of a more difficult and pleasing plate of shirred eggs in a carefully constructed nest of toast points.

I will never be the model of a Victorian angel. And, as my mother's daughter, I'm slowly coming to accept that. What's more, the deeper I read in the subject the more convinced I am that Mrs. Harland's friend was not alone in her unseemly outburst.

The clue I have for this resides in the class of invalid food called strengtheners. These were the dishes that were reserved for the later stages of an illness when the patient was on the mend, but still too weak to get out of bed. The purpose of these recipes falls into two distinct categories—to fatten the patient up if she's lost weight, and to revive flagging spirits. These dishes, full of carbohydrates, marrow meat, sugar, and, not infrequently, brandy or wine, are recorded in abundance, often with little goading asides to assure the care-giver that this is just the dish to push their patients up on their pins again. Recommended for convalescence from everything from the common cold to typhoid fever, these recipes sound as if the recorders—doctors and nurses or, like Mrs. Harland, no-nonsense household experts—feel called upon to shore up the reader's frayed nerves.

"It is at this time," Fannie Farmer states emphatically in *Food and Cookery for the Sick and Convalescent*, "when your patient, as well as yourself, will benefit most from a little amusement." She then goes on to give directions for something she calls Flower Pot Ice Cream—a serving of ice cream made to look like a flower blooming from a pot.

Not all of these dishes are visually amusing, but most of them do see that the patient continues on the road to recovery. Another good tip, from Dr. Alcinous B. Jamison, a noted internist at the turn of the century, is to begin slowly to exercise the patient. This may mean simply helping them from bed to a nearby chair or even to sit outside in the sunlight for an hour or two, the change of scenery often doing more good than all of modern medicine's miracles (this also provides an opportunity to completely air out the sickroom). He recommends a glass of red wine mixed with water at the afternoon and evening meals to help enrich the blood, stimulate the heart, and increase the appetite. Gentle massages and warm baths also help revive a sluggish circulatory system.

One more very sound piece of advice: As eager as you and the patient are for a full recovery, it cannot be hurried. If at all feasible, have the patient remain in bed—or at least sharply curtail activity—for a day longer than seems necessary. Continue treatment for a few days even after the symptoms of the illness are completely gone.

And for the care-giver? Do something that will brighten your waning spirits. Get away and give yourself a treat—take a walk, buy something nice, get a massage, or read a good book in the garden or in a quiet room of the house. When you come back, you won't be so tired, or nearly as peevish.

I HAVE DIVIDED THESE RECIPES into three sections. The first group is called restoratives, which are some of the oldest recipes I've come across, many dating from the eighteenth century. Serve them at the first turn toward health, when the stomach may still be weak but the appetite is beginning to revive. They are nutritious drinks (the precursor for modern supplements such as Ensure and Nutrical) and fare light enough to begin filling the stomach.

The second section features strengtheners, more filling dishes that begin to introduce more calories into the menu to build up stamina and combat weight loss.

The last section is comprised of, as Miss Farmer states, amusements—delicious treats to awaken the patient's dampened appetite for the final seduction back to health as well as several suggestions for a good night's sleep.

Restoratives

A RESTORATIVE JELLY

Makes enough for 1 day's serving

From the first edition of Mrs. Beeton's *Boston Cookbook*.

1 pound oxtails
1 pound beef shin bones
½ teaspoon coarse salt
Freshly ground pepper, optional

Have a large pot of boiling water on hand. Wash the oxtails very well, then blanch them in the pot of boiling water. Remove from the pot.

Cut the beef from the shin bone into small pieces. Place the beef and the oxtails in a small stockpot. Add 1 quart water and the salt. Bring the water to a boil, then lower the heat to a simmer. Cover the pot with a close-fitted lid and let cook for at least 7 hours, adding more water if necessary.

Strain the liquid through a fine-mesh sieve or a double layer of cheesecloth. Discard the bones and meat. Skim the liquid. Taste for seasoning (a small pinch of freshly ground pepper—not too much—may be added if you like) and pour into a bowl or mold and refrigerate until set. (This will come out not as firm as Jell-O, but rather like jam.) Serve at room temperature, or slightly warmed as a soup. This keeps only 2 days.

A STIMULATING JELLY

Makes 1 serving

Mrs. Farmer's entry—a little less straitlaced than Mrs. Beeton's.

¾ teaspoon unflavored gelatin
1 clove
1 cinnamon stick
½ cup strong beef stock (preferably homemade)
⅓ cup port wine

Soak the gelatin in ½ tablespoon cold water. In the top of a double boiler set over simmering water, heat the clove, cinnamon, beef stock, and wine for 10 minutes to warm through. Add the gelatin and stir to dissolve.

Strain the liquid through a fine-mesh sieve into a bowl or a pretty mold. Chill until set.

MAKING COD LIVER OIL PALATABLE

Makes 1 serving

Leave it to the French to figure out how to make something as revolting as cod liver oil taste reasonably good. Children today don't know how lucky they are that vitamin supplements have done away with the once common practice of forcing a teaspoon of this vile stuff down young throats. Cod liver oil has a very strong smell—and an equally strong fishy taste. But this method, devised by Alexis Soyer, uses fresh cod liver, with a very different (some might even consider luscious) flavor, which, nevertheless, delivers the vitamin wallop of straight oil.

1   pound fresh cod liver

2   pounds new white potatoes, peeled and partially steamed

Salt and freshly ground pepper, optional

In the top of a double boiler or steamer, arrange the liver over the potatoes. Steam until the liver is cooked all the way through, about 5 to 10 minutes.

Slice the liver into thin strips (to extract more of the oil) and arrange it beside the potatoes on a plate.

If the patient's stomach is not weak, the liver may be eaten with a little butter or anchovy sauce. The potatoes may be sprinkled with salt and a small grinding of fresh pepper if desired.

A VERY STRENGTHENING DRINK

Makes enough for 1 day

Another entry from Alexis Soyer is a sweet drink he recommends to be given at least 2 hours before the midday meal because it increases the appetite.

1 teaspoon pearl
  barley

Zest of 1 lemon,
pith removed

1 small cinnamon
  stick

Molasses, sugar, or
honey, optional

Place the pearl barley, 6 cups cold water, the lemon zest, and the cinnamon stick in a saucepan and bring to a boil. Simmer the barley until tender, about 15 minutes. Strain through a sieve and sweeten to taste with molasses, sugar, or honey if desired.

Sip slowly.

This may be stored in the refrigerator for two days but loses some of its flavor.

. . .

IRISH MOSS, also known as carrageen, is a stubby, purplish seaweed found on both the west coast of Ireland and on our eastern coast. It was once greatly relied on as a source of iron (my grandmother used to give it to her children every morning in dried little pieces that she called black candy!). It was also prized as a thickening agent for use in puddings and soups.

IRISH MOSS

Makes 4 small servings

This recipe is the most common preparation for Irish moss in cooking for the infirm—a pudding sometimes grandly called blanc mange. It was valued as a supplement. Mary Boland Pequignot says very sweetly, "It will form a tender jellylike pudding, which has an agreeable taste, resembling the odor of the sea," which, in itself, works wonders on a shut-in's tattered imagination.

⅓ cup dry Irish moss
1 quart milk
¼ cup sugar
    Light cream, optional

Soak the moss for ½ hour in warm water, washing each piece to remove any clinging sand.

    Wrap the moss in cheesecloth and immerse in the milk in the top of a double

boiler set over slowly simmering water. Cook
for 1 hour, being very careful the milk does
not become scorched.

Lift out the cheesecloth and squeeze to
drain all the liquid in the moss into the milk.
Add the sugar to the milk, then strain through
a fine sieve into a bowl. Cover with plastic
wrap directly on the surface of the milk (so
a scum does not form) and place in the
refrigerator until set.

The pudding will be a light jade color;
a serving suggestion by Miss Pequignot is to
surround the unmolded pudding with a
puddle of light cream. It will then resemble
an island in the middle of a moonlit sea.

INVALID'S TEA

Makes 1 serving

Even people who do not normally drink tea, will appreciate the more gentle effect of this brew over coffee. Most cookbooks maintain that tea made by the following method was extremely nourishing and a good afternoon stimulant for both patient and care-giver (though care-givers were admonished never to use the same spoon or dishes the patient used, or even to drink their tea in the sickroom, lest their cup become contaminated with airborne germs).

1 cup scalded milk	Bring the milk quickly to the scalding point in
1 level teaspoon of good loose tea	a small saucepan and pour it over the tea. Let the two infuse for 4 minutes, strain, and serve
Sugar, optional	with or without sugar to taste.

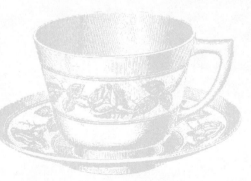

. . .

I SPENT A VERY nice day in the archives of the University of Pennsylvania's School of Nursing, digging through tiny little textbooks and manuals that hadn't been opened for years. One of the most useful books I found was the *Reference Hand Book for Nurses* (1905) by Amanda K. Beck, which listed all kinds of helpful tips and words of encouragement to professional nurses, especially for those out on their own in rural areas.

VEGETABLE SOUP FOR BABIES

Makes 4 servings

Despite the soup's name, I would also serve this to adults.

½ cup fresh, well-washed, finely chopped spinach

1 beet, peeled and finely chopped

1 carrot, peeled and finely chopped

Place the spinach, beet, carrot, and 4 cups water in a soup pot and bring to a boil. Lower the heat and cook for 1 hour or until the vegetables are tender.

Strain the soup through a fine sieve, pushing the soft vegetables against the mesh with the back of a spoon. Discard the vegetables.

The soup may be drunk from a baby bottle or, if the child is older, served in a bowl. For additional bulk, small pasta may be added.

OYSTER BROTH

Makes 1 serving

Dr. William W. Hall expressed the opinion that red pepper—just a little—strengthens weakened stomachs. I would think it would irritate them, but I'm partial to spicy things and after a few days of rather gentle food, or none at all, a little spark might be just the thing. This recipe, in particular, gives a nice jolt but I leave it to the reader's discretion whether to add red pepper here or anywhere else in these recipes.

12 oysters, finely
    chopped
¼ cup milk
⅛ teaspoon red
    pepper, optional

Put the oysters and 1 cup water in a large saucepan and bring to a boil. Simmer for 5 minutes until the oysters are cooked through. Just before serving, add the milk, and the red pepper if you like.

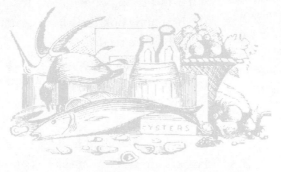

. . .

THE THREE NUTRITIOUS RECIPES that follow would be considered desserts anywhere outside the sickroom.

B A N A N A   F L I P

Makes 1 serving

This one comes from *The Scottish Bakehouse Cook Book*, which states, "If a person is on the mend, the food value in this dessert will send them further forward."

1 large egg white

⅛ teaspoon cream of tartar

½ cup heavy cream

1 banana

1 teaspoon fresh lemon juice

1 tablespoon sugar

Place the egg white, I teaspoon water, and the cream of tartar in a small saucepan. Stir together and cook over a very low flame, beating the mixture with a wire whisk, until the mixture reaches 160°F.

Pour into a bowl and whip until stiff peaks form. In another bowl, whip the cream until stiff peaks form, then fold the whites and cream together. Refrigerate.

Mash ¾ of the banana to a pulp; slice the rest and set aside.

Add the lemon juice to the mashed banana, then add the sugar and mix together. Fold in the egg white and cream. Place banana slices on the top.

EGG CREAM

Makes 4 small servings

Serve this on the breakfast tray or as a light pick-me-up in the afternoon.

2 large eggs, separated

2 level tablespoons sugar

Juice and grated zest of ½ lemon

Beat the yolks with the sugar until lightly lemon-colored. Add the lemon juice, zest, and 2 tablespoons water. Place in the top of a double boiler and cook over simmering water, stirring constantly, until the mixture begins to thicken and has reached 160°F. Remove from heat.

Whip the egg whites until thickened. Add to the yolk mixture and return the top of the double boiler to the simmering water. Cook the mixture, stirring gently, until it resembles thick cream; again, make sure the mixture reaches 160°F. Remove from heat, pour into individual serving cups, and cool in the refrigerator until set.

JUNKET EGGNOG

Makes 4 small servings

Miss Eliza Pitkin edited a book *(Invalid Cookery,* 1880) of invalid recipes from a Miss Julia Pye, who had served as a nurse in the Civil War. Eggnog was a staple of the sickroom, used to revive patients (and often tired visitors, as well). This particular recipe is a very dainty pudding, recommended for children, nursing mothers, and the elderly.

1 large egg, separated

2 level teaspoons sugar

2 teaspoons red wine

1 cup warm milk

½ teaspoon unflavored gelatin, softened in 1 teaspoon cold water

Nutmeg or cinnamon to taste, optional

Mix the yolk with the sugar and wine in a heavy saucepan, then add the egg white. Cook over very low heat, stirring constantly, until the mixture thickens and reaches 160°F. Remove from the heat and stir the milk into the egg mixture. Add the gelatin and stir until the gelatin has dissolved.

Pour at once into small glasses and grate a little nutmeg or cinnamon over the top if you like. Refrigerate until set.

WHITE CAUDLE

Makes about 3 servings

A caudle is defined as a hot drink with restorative powers. Dr. Robert Wallace Johnson recorded this one in 1819.

2 tablespoons Irish oatmeal

Pinch of mace

3 or 4 whole cloves

Grated zest from 1 medium lemon

1 cup good-quality white wine

Pinch of nutmeg, optional

Sugar, optional

Mix the oatmeal, 1 cup water, the mace, and cloves together in a medium saucepan. Bring to a boil and reduce to a simmer. Let cook for 15 minutes, stirring often. Add lemon zest and continue cooking for another 10 or 15 minutes or until all the liquid is absorbed.

Pour about ¼ cup of the warm oatmeal into a mug. Add about ⅓ cup wine and stir to mix. Add nutmeg and sugar to taste if desired. Sip leisurely. Repeat proportions for two additional servings as needed.

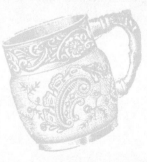

Strengtheners

ARROWROOT GRUEL

Makes 1 serving

Arrowroot gruel, by itself, contains little in the way of nutrients, but it was considered a very good stimulant to the appetite. *The Rumford Complete Cook Book*'s recipe suggests serving the gruel midmorning and again at teatime. I've seen many kinds of wine recommended for this gruel, including everything from a full-bodied red wine like Bordeaux to sweet wines, port, sherry, or brandy. Whatever you personally like will do.

1 tablespoon arrowroot

1 cup milk

Pinch of salt

Pinch of sugar

2 tablespoons brandy or wine

Mix the arrowroot with a little of the milk to form a smooth paste. Heat the rest of the milk in a small saucepan, then add the arrowroot paste and cook over low heat, stirring, for about 10 minutes. Add the salt and sugar to taste. Just before serving, add the brandy or wine.

EGG IN NEST

Makes 1 serving

I used to think of Fannie Farmer as a regular straitlaced Yankee girl. In the narrative that accompanies her remedy recipes, however, she reveals that there might have been flights of fancy and a sense of humor burbling within her tight stays. This recipe, found nowhere else in this type of cooking (the flower pot ice cream on page 148 is another unique Farmer invention), is a case in point.

1 large egg, separated

1 piece of toast

Preheat the oven to 350°F.

Beat the egg white until it forms stiff peaks. Dip the toast briefly in warm water, then place on a lightly buttered baking sheet. Mound the white over the toast. With the back of a tablespoon, make a shallow well in the center of the white, then carefully place the yolk in the depression.

Place the baking sheet in the middle of the oven and bake until the yolk is set and the whites are delicately brown, about 5 minutes—a little longer if you don't like a runny yolk.

SHIRRED EGG

Makes 1 serving

Just a lovely dish, especially for the first hunger pangs after a stomach virus; also good after a violent hangover has left you.

2 tablespoons soft bread crumbs (preferably homemade from good-quality bread)

½ tablespoon melted butter

1 large egg

Pinch of salt

Preheat the oven to 350°F.

Mix the crumbs and butter together and press them into the bottom of a custard cup or very small baking dish. Break the egg over the crumbs and sprinkle with a little salt. Sprinkle the top with any leftover crumbs and bake until the egg is set, about 5 to 10 minutes, depending on desired consistency.

·   ·   ·

EELS GIVE ME the willies. However, I do appreciate the considerable faith placed in them in invalid cooking. Eel meat, sweet and firm, is rich in vitamins A and D and an excellent source of protein—just what anyone would need to jump-start a sputtering system.

EEL BROTH

Makes 1 serving

I've come across several similar recipes but I'm going to use Alexis Soyer's, just because I trust him more and his recipes tend toward a bit more sophistication than the others. However, I do like the reassuring opinion that Dr. Robert Wallace Johnson attached to his recipe, in which he considered eel to be "superior to viper broth" (to which I can only add that I should hope so). Soyer believed that eel broth should be served in the fall (when young, tender specimens were caught), no matter if you were sick or not, to set you up for the winter.

1 small eel, skinned, washed, and sliced into serving pieces

1 teaspoon salt

1 sprig parsley

2 small onions, peeled, but left whole

1 clove

Place the pieces of eel in a small saucepan. Add the salt, parsley, onions, and clove and just enough water to cover the meat. Bring to a simmer, skimming the scum and fat that will rise to the surface. Cook until tender, about ½ hour. Remove from heat.

Pour the liquid through a fine-mesh sieve placed over a serving bowl. With the back of a spoon, press the meat against the mesh to extract any juices.

Serve only the broth, a teaspoon at a time, for very weak patients (the eel meat will be too rich for their stomachs). For more robust constitutions or to be used as a tonic, the fish can be served on the side or added to the broth.

SOUP MEAGRE

Makes 4 servings

While this seems to be nothing more than a thin onion soup, the magic bullet here is the addition of vinegar at the end. At one time vinegar was thought to stimulate the appetite, while also being an effective germ killer—sort of an internal antibacterial agent. The egg yolks make this a fairly nutritious little bowl of soup. It comes highly recommended by Dr. Robert Wallace Johnson, who reported in his book that it revived many of his patients during the great cholera epidemic of 1810.

½ pound (2 sticks) sweet butter

6 medium onions, sliced into thin rounds

2 celery stalks, diced

1 sprig parsley

2 tablespoons flour

½ cup torn pieces of hard (stale) bread

1 teaspoon freshly ground pepper

Pinch of mace, optional

2 large egg yolks, broken and stirred

1 teaspoon cider vinegar

Melt the butter in a deep stew pot, then add the onions. Cook over low heat until transparent. Add the celery and parsley and cook another 15 minutes, then sprinkle the flour over the vegetables and stir to blend. Add 4 cups boiling water, the stale bread, pepper, and mace if desired. Bring to a slow boil and cook for ½ hour. Just before serving, stir in the egg yolks and vinegar and let simmer until the yolks are set. Pour into a bowl and serve.

STEWED MACARONI

Makes 4 small servings

A pleasingly warm dish, stewed macaroni is just the thing when your stomach has been wracked with pain. The macaroni is melting soft, surrounded by a thin sauce of milk; it has the effect of making your stomach feel as if it is wrapped up in a comforting quilt. Serve only a little at first, maybe just a cup, then increase the amount to a full serving. This keeps in the refrigerator for three days.

1 tablespoon butter	Bring I quart salted water and the butter
½ pound macaroni	to a boil in a medium saucepan. Add the
1 tablespoon flour	macaroni and cook until soft. Do not drain.
1 cup warm milk	Remove from the heat and stir in the flour
1 tablespoon honey or brown sugar, optional	until the lumps are gone. Add the warm milk and stir until you have the consistency of
½ cup milk or cream, optional	melted butter.

Return the pan to low heat and continue cooking, stirring constantly, for about another 20 minutes. Three minutes before serving, you may add a sweetener or the milk or cream if desired.

SCRAPED BEEF SANDWICH

Makes 1 serving

This is known in my house as a "going back to school sandwich." When my kids have been sick and they see me making one, they know there's school the following day. The original recipe does not call for Tabasco; in fact, it's just the beef and a very small amount of salt and pepper. But my children like spicy things, and the hot pepper sauce adds a little zing that is so desperately needed after days of a fairly bland diet.

¼ pound very lean cold cooked steak
Tabasco
Salt and pepper
2 pieces of toast

Remove all the fat from the meat. With the blade of a knife, scrape the meat pulp from the fiber into a small bowl. (An easier method, and less tedious, is to chop the meat in a food processor, using the metal blade. The meat will be just a little rougher.) Season to taste with the Tabasco, salt, and pepper.

Spread the meat on one slice of toast, buttered or plain. Top with the other slice of toast, cut into strips, and serve.

Amusements

There's absolutely no reason in the world why you or anyone else in the house can't enjoy these dishes as well. A few of them require a small amount of alcohol—2 tablespoons, tops—but enough to give a kick. If you don't drink, or don't think the patient should, just omit the liquor.

ORANGE SHERBET

Makes 4 servings

This sherbet is very refreshing to a feverish patient right after the fever breaks or for everyone on a warm day. I found the original recipe in Mary Boland Pequignot's book, *A Handbook of Invalid Cooking*, but I've added the bit about freezing the sherbet in an orange skin just because it's fun.

1 cup freshly squeezed orange juice (about 4 oranges)	Cut the oranges in half and carefully squeeze the juice from each half. Scoop as much pulp as you can from the interiors and save the 4 nicest halves.

1 tablespoon
  unflavored gelatin

1 cup sugar

¼ cup freshly
  squeezed lemon
  juice (about 1 large
  lemon)

2 tablespoons brandy

Dissolve the gelatin in I cup boiling water. When it's completely dissolved, add the orange juice, sugar, lemon juice, and brandy. Stir to dissolve the sugar. Let the mixture cool.

When the mixture is cool, pour into an ice-cream maker and freeze according to the manufacturer's directions. Scoop the finished sherbet into the reserved orange skins. Cover with plastic wrap and place in freezer until ready to serve.

PEACH FOAM

Makes 1 serving

Miss Pequignot really drools over this recipe. Not only does she un-characteristically proclaim it to be delicious but she recommends that it "may be eaten *ad liberum* by the invalid."

1 large egg white
3 or 4 very ripe peaches
½ cup confectioners' sugar

Stir the egg white and 1 teaspoon water together in a small heavy saucepan. Cook over very low heat, whisking constantly, until the white reaches 160°F. Remove from heat.

Peel and cut the peaches into small pieces. Place them in the bowl of a food processor fitted with the metal blade (a blender will also do nicely). Add the sugar and the egg white and process until the mixture is smooth and velvety.

COFFEE CREAM

Makes 4 servings

As may be self-evident, try this as an antidote to fatigue—whether from ordinary life or the rigors of fighting germs.

1 packet unflavored gelatin

½ cup freshly brewed strong coffee

½ cup sugar

1¼ cups heavy cream, whipped

2 tablespoons coffee-flavored liqueur

Soften the gelatin in ¼ cup cold water in the top of a double boiler. Add the coffee and set over simmering water until the gelatin dissolves. Add the sugar and stir until it is dissolved. Remove from the heat and strain into a bowl.

Place the bowl in another bowl filled with ice. When the mixture begins to thicken (or as Miss Pequignot notes, "or is about the consistency of molasses on a warm day"), gently fold in the whipped cream and liqueur until everything is well mixed (it will be a light mocha color). Turn into serving dishes or a pretty glass bowl and place in the refrigerator for at least 3 hours, or until set.

FANNIE FARMER'S FLOWER POT ICE CREAM

Makes 1 serving

All I can say is that, as silly as this may seem, there is a time and a place in the sickroom for shenanigans. It usually comes about the third day after your charge begins to really feel better but may be a little depressed at how tired and weak he or she still feels. Late afternoon seems to be the time of most distress—when night is coming on and the patient may be just a little disoriented. This is the perfect moment to serve up a bit of comfort and delight.

¼ to ½ cup good ice cream in the patient's favorite flavor (the amount depends on the size of the flower pot, so don't choose a very big pot), softened

1 tablespoon Dutch-process cocoa

1 tablespoon grated bittersweet chocolate

1 flower with a firm stem

Line the sides and bottom of a small flower pot (a clay or ceramic seedling pot is perfect) with wax paper, trimming the paper to fit just to the pot's rim. Fill the pot with the ice cream. Cover with plastic wrap and place in the freezer until firm.

When ready to serve, take the pot out of the freezer. Remove the plastic wrap and sift the cocoa over the surface of the ice cream, then sprinkle the chocolate over the cocoa. Wash the flower's stem, then stick it in the middle of the ice cream. Serve at once.

Sleep Aids

The following are specifically recommended to combat sleepless-
ness—a common side-effect toward the end of an illness. The first
two are light and very boozy recipes. I have given the first one, made
with sherry, to my children with no adverse effect. The second one, a
proper eggnog, I reserve for drinking adults. The third direction is actually physical therapy and works very well, not just for the sick but
for anyone experiencing restlessness due to stress.

VELVET CREAM

Makes 4 servings

1 package unflavored
   gelatin
¼ cup best sherry
1 teaspoon lemon
   juice
½ cup sugar
1¼ cups milk or heavy
   cream

Soften the gelatin in ¼ cup cold water in the
top of a double boiler. Stir in the sherry and
place the pan over simmering water. Stir until
the gelatin dissolves, then add the lemon juice
and sugar, stirring well. When the sugar has
dissolved, pour the mixture into a bowl and
set it over ice, stirring until it thickens. Pour in
the milk or cream and continue stirring until
the mixture thickens further. Place the bowl in
the refrigerator and chill until set.

EGGNOG

Makes 1 serving

Make sure the egg is very fresh.

1   large egg,
    separated
⅔ cup cold milk
1   tablespoon sugar
    Pinch of salt
2   tablespoons rum or
    brandy
⅛ teaspoon cream of
    tartar

Beat the yolk in a heavy saucepan until it's a light yellow color, then add the milk, sugar, and salt. Cook over low heat, stirring constantly, until the mixture lightly coats the back of a wooden spoon and has reached 160°F. Remove from the heat and place the saucepan in a bowl filled with ice water to cool. Stir in the liquor and beat until smooth.

Place in the refrigerator while you beat the egg white. (You can hold the mixture at this point until you're ready to serve.)

Put the egg white, 1 teaspoon water, and the cream of tartar in another heavy saucepan. Cook over low heat, beating the mixture with a wire whisk, until it reaches 160°F. Remove from heat and pour into a medium bowl. Beat the egg white until stiff.

When you are ready to serve, fold the beaten egg white thoroughly into the yolk mixture. Serve immediately.

. . .

IN TIMES PAST, nursing was sometimes regarded as a job for the disreputable. Good women, it was thought, would either be too squeamish or modest to take on the ghastly duties the profession required. Florence Nightingale had to fight this battle, especially as an unmarried woman and therefore, presumably, a sexually innocent woman. She must have seen everything in the Crimean War. She didn't flinch, but when it came time for massages—a treatment often advised by doctors—she demanded that more than one nurse always be present in the room and that the massage be administered through a shielding sheet so that her nurses would not be accused of any indecent behavior.

A RUB FOR RESTLESSNESS

Makes about 1 pint

Fortunately, times have changed. Today, this rub can be given as it should: the patient undressed or just covered with a sheet. There is nothing like it to put the body at ease. This rub recipe comes from Miss Eliza Pitkin, who very sensibly warns that it is only to be used on patients free of skin rashes or open sores (watch out for painful bed sores) which may become aggravated both by the ingredients and the rubbing.

1 cup rubbing
alcohol

1 tablespoon Epsom
salts

1 ounce aromatic
ammonia or
perfumed oil
(see Note)

Mix together I cup water, the rubbing alcohol, Epsom salts, and ammonia or oil. Shake well in a securely sealed bottle.

To Massage: Pour a little of the liquid on your hands before rubbing on the body. Gently rub each limb, the torso, neck, and temples, until a pleasant glow appears on the skin.

Note: There are many different kinds of oil on the market today, a lot of them with very specific properties. I am not a great believer in most of the benefits ascribed to aromatherapy or other New Age kinds of treatments, though I think they're certainly pleasant and that in itself is a recommendation. Choose an oil with a scent that is personally pleasing to you or the patient. Just make sure it doesn't have an overpowering smell. Remember that the sick are often more sensitive to smell and other sensory experiences.

What to Do with an Aching Body

**Muscle Aches,
Pains, Injuries**

Some people go through their whole lives suffering little more than minor cuts and bruises. Others are not as lucky. The prognosis becomes apparent early on in the rough and tumble years of childhood when the invulnerable and the accident-prone begin to reveal themselves. The brave adventures and stupid stunts of adolescence and the death-defying acts of teenagers leave some without a scar while others learn the insides of emergency rooms like their own homes.

I am in the latter category. Sprained muscles, swollen joints, burns, and bruises are a regular part of my life. My bones are host to an array of metal posts and pins. Most of the time, however, even the most serious of my accidents are relatively minor, quickly dealt with and healed; but their frequency is a cause of considerable terror and amusement for my family.

One could say I'm rash, that I do things without planning, much less thinking. One could also say, as my family frequently does, that I am impatient and a little absentminded. It's all true. It's my nature—I like to do a lot of things at once.

The up side of all these misadventures is that I've gotten pretty good at tending to wounds and remaining level-headed when accidents happen. Blood and guts, oddly jutting bones, don't faze me. And I usually don't collapse until the crisis is well over. I like to think that all my mishaps have served a good purpose.

Miss Nightingale once stated, in her usual emphatic style, that "Every woman, or at least almost every woman, in England has, at one time or another in her life, charge of the personal health of somebody . . . in other words, every woman is a nurse." I would amend her statement now to include everybody, male and female, who has to nurse someone at some time in life, even if it's only themselves. Some people, because of their nature and circumstances, just get more practice than others.

Long before hospitals were built kitchens were the nearest emergency ward. A standard inventory of the first-aid kitchen cabinet included clean strips of cotton for binding wounds, a thermometer, an enema bag, bottles of aromatic spirit of ammonia, baking soda, sweet spirit of nitre, a disinfectant (typically chloride of lime, carbolic acid, and especially phenol sodique), a lubricating ointment, Epsom salts, boric acid, and a deodorizer such as rose or lavender water. Alongside these basics would be some patent medicines—such as Humphrey Remedies—and a few herbal mixtures.

Many other first-aid supplies came directly from the pantry shelves. While old first-aid techniques are decidedly low tech, a lot of them are just as effective, such as those that follow.

THE FIRST HOME REMEDY I ever learned of came from my pediatrician; it was verified by a friend's mother from Poland (who came to America alone at the age of 15 after being freed from a concentration camp). The remedy is for earaches and is meant to be used until you can get to a doctor. It's especially useful for babies who are very susceptible to getting ear infections.

EMERGENCY EARACHE CURE

Makes 1 treatment

This recipe comes from the Van Rensselaer family, an old, wealthy New York clan mentioned earlier. I have adapted the directions for a modern stove.

1 tablespoon olive oil, the purer the better

Heat the oil in a small saucepan over low heat until **tepid—NOT HOT** (test on the back of your wrist as you would for a baby's bottle). It

must be just warm—any hotter and you run
the risk of perforating the ear). Using a
dropper, squeeze a small drop in the ear.
Cover the ear with a warm towel and lie still
for a few minutes.

THE ONION CURE

Makes 1 treatment

The Van Rensselaer girls claim this recipe cures earaches only sometimes, and while it seems the onion itself has very little to do with its
effectiveness, I'm inclined to recommend its use coupled with the previous recipe. The onion will keep the small drop of oil warm as it
gently presses on the inflamed organ, which will then temporarily relieve pain.

1 onion cut in half
to the size of
patient's ear

Preheat the oven to 350°F.
    Gently roast each half of the onion until
nicely warm but not too soft. Remove from
the oven and wrap in a warm, clean linen
handkerchief. Press against the ear.

. . .

THE VAN RENSSELAERS put much more faith in their cure for hearing difficulties. The main ingredient here is foxglove, a very beautiful flowering perennial. Both its flowers and the leaves, have been used for medicinal purposes since ancient times and continue to be of great value in our time, especially for heart disease. However, even if you have lots of the flowers growing in your garden, do not take it upon yourself to prepare anything with them that you will ingest. Unless you know precisely what you are doing, you may actually end up poisoning yourself. Parts of the plant (in greater or lesser degree depending on the different varieties) contain digitoxin, an extremely potent drug that acts directly on the heart.

This recipe, however, is harmless. I've tried it out on my father-in-law, a patient, good-natured man whose ears have been blasted to pulp by years of being a disk jockey and listening to ear drum splitting decibels through headphones. His testimony is that he did hear a little clearer in the time he used what I gave him—about a week's worth. As soon as he stopped, though, despite the Van Rensselaer's claim, his deafness returned.

HEARING DIFFICULTIES

Makes enough for 2 night treatments

2 or 3 fresh
leaves from a
2-year-old
foxglove plant

2 tablespoons
brandy

Process the leaves in a juicer. If you don't have a juicer, gently shred the leaves. Put them in a bowl, and pour about ½ cup of boiling water over them (just enough to wet the leaves). Let steep for 1 hour, pressing the leaves with the back of a spoon to extract as much juice as possible, then drain, reserving the juice and discarding the leaves. You need 2 tablespoons of juice.

Pour the juice into a small bowl and mix with the brandy (if you have less than 2 tablespoons of juice, adjust the amount of brandy to use equal parts liquor to juice).

Place a single small drop in each ear. Soak a bit of lint or a cotton ball in the remaining juice and pack it in the ear. Keep cloth or cotton ball in the ear overnight, removing it in the morning. Repeat as often as possible, until deafness is cured.

. . .

ANOTHER INFALLIBLE CURE from the Van Rensselaers is for toothaches. The main ingredient is Peruvian bark, also known as red bark or Jesuits' powder. You can find it in most health food stores. Peruvian bark is an astringent in the powder form; in its liquid form (also available) it is a very good tonic, useful in the cure of drunkenness and hangovers. (Use too much, though, and it will give you a violent headache all by itself.)

This cure was also used by the Van Rensselaer household as a mouthwash, to preserve the teeth and gums. (It has a very powerful kick to it, which on some mornings may be of value but should, perhaps, be avoided if you have to present yourself in any dignified context.)

INFALLIBLE CURE FOR TOOTHACHE

Makes 1½ quarts

½ cup Peruvian bark, finely powdered

2 cups best quality brandy

2 cups rose water

Mix the bark, brandy, and rose water together in a glass or earthenware jug. Let sit for 24 hours, then pour into a bottle with a tight-fitting lid.

Take 1 mouthful every morning. Hold in mouth for 5 minutes, concentrating liquid on painful spot.

As a mouthwash, gently swish the liquid over teeth and gums every morning.

. . .

A SIMPLER TOOTHACHE CURE comes from Dr. William Hall. He swore by the following, which relies on pressure-point therapy as much as on its one ingredient. It's rather messy and smelly, but I think not unpleasantly so, especially since a toothache makes it rare that you'll wish to be in company.

A TOOTHACHE REMEDY

Makes 1 treatment

1 very fresh young horseradish root

Grate about I tablespoon of horseradish from the root. Apply directly to the wrist over the pulse point, binding it in place with a clean linen handkerchief tightly enough to feel some pressure and heat from the root but not enough to cut circulation. Leave in place until the heat is gone.

. . .

ANOTHER POULTICE with a long list of testimonials from medieval herbal books straight on down to modern medical practices is this one using flax and mustard seeds. It works exceedingly well but it's rather smelly—but then many commercial alternatives aren't exactly perfumed, either. This particular version of the poultice comes from Margaret J. Thompson's *Food for the Sick and Well.*

A POULTICE

Makes 1 treatment

1 cup flaxseeds
1 cup mustard seeds

Crush the flax and mustard seeds with a pestle and mortar (a food processor, using the metal blade, will also suffice) until finely crushed. Add ¼ cup hot water, stirring until a thick paste is formed (add more hot water if necessary).

Spread the paste on half of a piece of old muslin or double-thick cheesecloth in a thick layer. Fold the other half over the paste.

Place the prepared cloth in a hot basin or bowl. Let the poultice sit for a few minutes to absorb some of the bowl's heat—but not too hot or it will burn the patient's skin! Apply the cloth directly to the affected area, letting it stay in place until all the heat has evaporated.

✺ FOR CURING CRACK'D SKIN ✣

*(This recipe is included for its historical relevance only.
It is **not** recommended for modern-day use.)*

For a sprain, the Van Rensselaers used a mixture of vinegar and NATS Foot oil or rendered animal fat, smeared on a piece of flannel and heated to a high temperature, then wrapped around the injury. This helped only because of the heat. But another paste made, of all things, with buttercups is a sweeter remedy in the removal of warts, canker sores, and healing all kinds of blisters, as well as giving relief from the physical symptoms of gout (swollen joints). Here is the original recipe from 1834, recorded in a Van Rensselaer's hand. It makes about 1 day's treatment, depending on how many buttercups you've gathered.

"Take a root call'd Crows foot (common buttercups, flower, stem, leaves and roots), dried and steep'd like tea. Wash three or four times a day till well—amen."

I consider the amen part to be an essential direction for the recovery. For swollen joints, make a paste of the leaves—you'll need to gather a rather large amount of buttercups which may, in itself, swell a joint or two, but there are worse ways to spend a day.

. . .

LONG SOAKS in a nice warm bath that is infused with several different ingredients are also wonderful cures, not only for aching, swollen
joints but for broken hearts and collapsed psyches. Although most soaking recipes will do for just about any ailment, I've come across a few
that are reserved for special situations.

Such as growing pains. I have found that the following, recommended by Dr. Robert Wallace Johnson, works as a miraculous water
treatment to combat foul adolescent-teenage moods (anywhere from
ten to sixteen years of age, but by no means exclusively). Girls, I hear,
are easier than boys to lure into a full tub, but once you have persuaded
them to try it out, both sexes emerge as clean as the infants they once
were. And almost as sweet-tempered.

A COURSE FOR GROWING PAINS

Makes 1 treatment

1 cup freshly picked
   catnip and
   peppermint
½ cup sea salt or
   Epsom salts
1 cup cider vinegar

Fill a long basin (tub) with hot water and add
a large handful of the leaves of freshly picked
catnip and peppermint. Salt dried from the
sea is also useful in this preparation (add a
handful), as well as new cider vinegar—about
1 cup. Soak until the water has cooled. Rub
the skin to a glow before a bright fire.

. . .

THIS SOAK IS RESERVED for rashes, especially those caused by plants, allergies, or nerves. It comes from the Amish. In cases concerning nerves, it is further recommended to add lavender blossoms and to rest in the water, like Blanche Dubois, for as long as the world will let you.

FOR RASHES

Makes 1 treatment

2 tablespoons sage leaves (fresh are better; dried will do)

1 cup aloe vera (available in health food stores as a liquid)

1 cup apple cider vinegar

Add all the ingredients to a bath drawn with very warm water. Soak for at least 10 minutes at a time, longer if possible.

. . .

SCIATICA CAN BE greatly relieved with this soak. The use of a towel may seem unusual but it cushions the injury and feels good against the skin.

SCIATICA SOAK

Makes 1 treatment

1 tablespoon grated fresh ginger

1 cup apple cider vinegar

Lay a towel or soft cotton on the bottom of the tub and draw a shallow bath of warm water (enough water to cover the legs). Add the ginger and vinegar, stirring with your hands to mix well with the water. Soak for 15 minutes, making sure the legs and buttocks rest on the cloth and that the muscles are as relaxed as possible.

Cuts and Abrasions

The older literature on the treatment of cuts and abrasions reads somewhat like old penny novels, with vivid descriptions of wounds caused by musket balls, axes, arrowheads, knives, iron nails, and scythes.

When a wound occurs, consider its location and how deep it is. Those that are on or near arteries require pressure to stop the bleeding (the blood will come out in spurts and be bright red). Apply firm pressure just above and below the cut until the bleeding stops. Alternatively, apply a tight bandage or tourniquet.

If the wound is not too deep (no stitches required), the most important treatment is to clean it out. Let it bleed a little, to help clean out any foreign particles, then seal the wound with an antiseptic. A good modern antibiotic ointment always beats out old preparations, but if you don't have any around, the next best things are what Dr. Robert Wallace Johnson relied upon in 1819. He suggested using the following in order of his preference:

Cobwebs: Apply directly over the wound, packing them into the cut. Cobwebs are mentioned almost universally as a wound sealer, but until I tried them out I did not believe they would work. I was also, frankly, squeamish about the whole thing. But for the sake of this book, I ventured out into the garden (Dr. Robert Wallace Johnson recommended the garden [as opposed to attics and basements where the cobwebs might be contaminated by dirt and dust] and early morning as the optimum gathering time). Cobwebs are, indeed, gossamer things and, at first, it looked as if I had nothing in my hands, but as I went along, a sticky pearly substance began to materialize. The harvest I gathered in my small garden amounted to a tiny ball, enough to seal a gash I made in my hand while putting together a bookcase. I packed in the web and covered it with a bandage; two days later, the wound was clear, almost healed.

Onion: Mix the juice of one onion, with a little apple cider vinegar. Soak cotton balls in the solution and apply to the wound.

Cayenne: Sprinkle cayenne pepper over the wound. Aside from being an antiseptic, cayenne coagulates blood quickly. However, if the skin becomes irritated, suspend use.

Sage Leaves: Lay fresh leaves over the area.

FOR FRESH WOUNDS

Makes enough for 2 small treatments or 1 large one

The Van Rensselaers used oak gall—larvae of different insects on oak trees. Gall is one of the most effective natural coagulants and, thankfully, is now available in a powder form in most health food stores.

1 tablespoon powdered gall

4 tablespoons benzoate lard

Make a plaster by mixing the gall with the lard and apply directly to wound.

· · ·

WHILE THERE ARE many effective cures for animal and insect bites, the following are my favorites for a variety of reasons. The first I've actually tried—successfully. The next two I hope I never have to use, and the last just amuses me and I keep it in my head, often repeating it to myself like a song.

FOR BEE STINGS

Makes 1 treatment

Marion Harland, that sensible housewife, recorded this in *The New Common Sense in the Household*.

1 tablespoon wheat germ 2 tablespoons honey	Mix together to form a paste and rub over the sting. It will relieve the itching and take down the swelling.

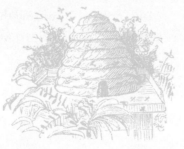

TO CURE BITES

These two cures for snakebites—the first for the common snake and the second for rattlesnakes—are taken from *Information for Everybody: An Invaluable Collection of About Eight Hundred Practical Recipes,* published in 1866. This book was something like the *Joy of Cooking*—it seemed that everybody, from Boston households to wagon trains, kept a copy. The first treatment for the nonpoisonous snake is said to be an Indian cure and is very simple (as long as you can quickly find this one herb).

◆§ COMMON SNAKEBITE ξ◆

(This recipe is included for its historical relevance only.
*It is **not** recommended for modern-day use.)*

Makes 1 treatment

Apply finely crumbled catnip to the bite of a snake. Leave in place overnight. Add more catnip the next day until the bite is gone.

⤳ RATTLESNAKE BITE ⤶

*(This recipe is included for its historical relevance only.
It is **not** recommended for modern-day use.)*

The rattlesnake treatment is a little more elaborate, since the snake is considerably more dangerous.

> Make a plaster of salt and I large egg yolk
> and smooth over the fang marks. If this
> doesn't work, try adding raw onions—finely
> grated—on top of the yolk mixture. Let dry.

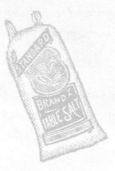

❧ A CURE FOR THE BITE ❧
OF A MAD DOG

(This recipe is included for its historical relevance only.)

My favorite cure by far (except, of course, for the nymphomaniac cure on page 38), is this one. It's literate, fun, and places great dependence on the power of faith (and I by no means recommend it as a cure!). It comes from the notebook of Mrs. Martha Bradley (late of Bath) in her book *British House-wife or the Cook, Housekeeper and Gardener's Companion* (1770).

> **Affrat, Frasret, Frasset;** give the person or animal one of these words written in their order as they stand on three mornings successively.
>
> *(Modern Translation:* Each morning, write one of these words on a piece of paper *[affrat* on the first morning, then *frasret,* then *frasset].* The person [or animal] is then supposed to relieve him/itself on the paper. Very important: The urine must be the first of the morning.)
>
> Hard to say, but, one hopes this is one treatment.

The Change in Seasons

Spring and Winter Tonics

Every August, my grandmother insisted on being taken to the Atlantic Ocean. My father, a man she did not like very much because he had a college degree, took off from work, packed us into the Rambler, and we all headed for the beach. ("A man with that much learning never amounts to good," my grandmother told my mother often enough for her four-year-old granddaughter to remember vividly how the words traversed the thicket of her deep brogue.) While my sister, brother, and I cavorted in the waves, my mother huddled under a large striped umbrella to protect her fair skin. My father waded into the surf to cast out a fishing line. And my grandmother rolled down her thick black stockings, pinned her voluminous dress around her knees, and wandered down the beach with a galvanized bucket to collect seaweed. When the bucket was full, she was ready to go home. She sat down in the car and waited until we packed up sandy towels and blankets. She hugged the bucket on her lap the whole way up the New Jersey Turnpike while her grandchildren, dazed, freckled, and burnt by the sun, collapsed against her soft body, and my parents, sitting close together in the front seat, smoked endless cigarettes and listened to the songs on the radio.

The next morning, we'd wake up to the sound of pounding in the backyard. My grandmother, a vigorous woman despite the dementia stealing up fast, sat on the back stoop with the bucket of seaweed at her feet. She took a few strands out, smoothed them across the cement steps, then mashed them with a small rock she had found and washed for the purpose. After the nodes were crushed, she dropped the flattened seaweed in another bucket filled with fresh water and repeated the same process with the other strands until all the seaweed was transferred to the new bucket. Over the following days, she continued to drain the bucket and add new water, each time running a hard stream of water over the seaweed. The air around the corner of the patio where the bucket sat became saturated with a sweet salty rot. Sometimes, when my grandmother was away from her watch, I'd plunge my hand under the cool brackish water, wiggling my fingers like frisky caterpillars through the silky strands floating just below the surface. After a week, the bucket was emptied into a large soup pot and placed on the back burner. Every other week of the year my mother ruled the kitchen, but for the next few days she would not step across the linoleum threshold. Through the screened windows, the house began to expel a tart humid breath, and by the time my father came home from work, my mother was ready to escape. As long as the seaweed bubbled on the stove, we went to drive-in movies, consumed the contents of the concession stands, thrilled at illicit steak sandwiches and pizza. My mother for once did not worry that we were not eating enough from the essential food groups to keep us alive. By the time we got back home, my grandmother would be asleep on a chair before the stove, a green-tinged wooden spoon cradled loosely in her open palms.

This was how my grandmother made her winter tonic, a magic potion to ward off germs and other lurking malicious spirits. Every September since then, a bitter taste creeps over my tongue. I think my mother tried to shield us from this experience, but her strong-willed mother always won. I can still see the tiny sterling silver sugar spoon with an Irish harp on the handle coming toward my lips. My brother, an enormous, sweet-tempered baby in my mother's lap, spits the stuff violently from his mouth and receives a sharp smack on the back of his hand. My sister, smart and independent, says she'll take hers with a sugar cube. My mother mixes hers in a cup of tea. My father and grandmother swig their doses straight from the bottle, my father twisting his face into a rubbery grimace to make his children laugh.

This is my idea of a tonic—a strange elixir, often rank and foul, that somehow purifies and prepares the body for a new season. It is an age-old tradition among most of the world's population to produce specific brews from native plants and roots just for the fall and spring.

The spring elixirs were formulated to purge the blood and organs of sluggish waste (the by-products of heavy food and inactivity) so the body would regain its strength for the hardworking summer months. The fall's concoctions were devised to store energy and warmth, a way of banking the body's resources for winter's severe conditions and inevitable shortages.

I really don't know what my grandmother's seaweed tonic did beyond contributing a lot of iodine to our systems, but I do know that my family, the children in particular, were annoyingly healthy. My brother and sister never missed a day of grade school (some behavioral absences ruined my record), and my mother flies through health crises that would send another to her deathbed. My father's poor health record—his one big cold a year—was blamed by my grandmother on all the germs spewing from the pages of the books he read.

Alexis Soyer pointed out that most mammals digest particular herbs and grasses at different times of the year. He observed that many of the animals on his farm outside of Paris wandered on their own into meadows where many wild herbs grew. "They do this as if beckoned by a common voice to do so. I do not pretend to say that it would suit persons in every malady, but I respect that this is a most useful and refreshing practice for the blood." (*Soyer's Cookery Book*, 1854). By late August, his fat and robust cows, dogs, and sheep, their hides and fur grown dense, their movements more languid, began to eat less grass and more grain. His geese were the exception. They continued to hawk and bray for more and more of everything. "Stupid creatures," Soyer chided. "But then, perhaps, they understand the Noël feast is fast approaching."

The tonics for spring are, by and large, based on young, tender herbs. Not only are the plants generally tastier in this innocent state but they are chock-full of vitamins and minerals. If it can't be *scientifically* proven that they purify the system, they certainly hit it with a vitamin wallop. One of the best is recorded by Soyer as being popular with the peasants around his estate, who administered it not only to themselves but, he noted, fed it to their animals, mixing it in with the slop.

A FRENCH TONIC

Makes 1 day's treatment

40 young sorrel leaves

1 small new green cabbage, chopped

10 young chervil sprigs

1 teaspoon coarse salt

1 teaspoon sweet butter

Bring 4 cups water to a boil in a large saucepan and add the sorrel, cabbage, chervil, salt, and butter. Lower the heat to a very slow simmer and let cook for no more than 4 minutes.

Strain the liquid through a fine sieve into a bowl, pressing the leaves and herbs with the back of a wooden spoon to extract all the liquid. Discard the leaves and store the liquid in a stone jug.

> Drink (hot or cold) 1 quart a day for
> 1 week. (Make a new batch as needed.)
> This is also a very good liquid to give to
> convalescents—dilute with water (about
> 2 cups more water to the same quantity
> of herbs).

. . .

A FRIEND in Vermont sent me a tonic that is somewhat similar but calls for an immense gathering of meadow plants. She received a bottle of it from her neighbor—a woman she refers to as "Ethan Frome's wife." She sips at this brew through the first warm weeks in May and claims that it is the only thing that has kept her alive. That's an awful lot to declare for what is really a simple drink, but I'm betting that, with the amount of liquor the recipe calls for, she must—at the very least—experience a lighter spirit during those sweet May days.

THE MEADOW TONIC

Fills two 750-ml wine bottles

15 meadow plants, leaves and roots, gathered while they're still young (see Note)

Clean the meadow plants under a strong stream of water. Shred the leaves and dice the roots. Place the leaves and roots in an earthenware or glass jug or bowl and pour

1   bottle good white
    wine
¼ cup honey
1¼ cups good fruit
    brandy (homemade
    is best)

the wine over the plants. Cover with a cloth
and let steep for at least 3 days, stirring
occasionally.

Remove the cover and pour the wine and
plants into a stainless steel saucepan. Bring to
a boil over medium heat. Remove from heat
and strain the liquid through a fine-mesh sieve
into a bowl. Press the leaves and roots with
the back of a spoon to extract any remaining
juices. Discard the leaves and roots.

While the liquid is still hot, add the
honey, stirring until it dissolves. Let cool
completely. Add the fruit brandy and stir.

Pour the liquid into a wine bottle or a
plastic milk carton and set it in a dark cool
place until the following spring. It can be used
directly from the container.

Note: Plants to gather: licorice, milk thistle, yellow dock, wild thyme,
burdock root, dandelion, beets, parsnip, carrots, lovage, chicory root,
wild yam root, nettle leaves, violet leaves and flowers, mint, mustard
greens, chickweed, watercress, wild arugula.

. . .

ANOTHER WILD MIXTURE was recommended by Dr. John Fothergill, who listed the following soup as a great benefit to those who have spent the winter convalescing. With English pride, he noted that, "while it is fashionable to partake of European waters, I have found this soup, made from Our Native Specimens to be of more benefit to the weaken[ed] constitution."

A TONIC SOUP

Makes 4 to 6 servings

2 sweet onions, sliced

2 fresh burdock roots

¼ cup yellow dock root

½ cup dandelion roots

1 fresh young beet

1 young parsnip

1 new potato, in medium dice

2 young carrots

2 ounces kelp

1 lovage stalk, chopped

1 cup chopped dandelion leaves

1 cup chopped yellow dock greens

1 large garlic clove, diced

Put 6 cups water in a large stockpot and add the onions, roots, beet, parsnip, potato, carrots, kelp, and lovage. Bring to a simmer over low heat and cook for about 30 minutes, or until the roots and vegetables are tender.

Add the greens and garlic and simmer only a few minutes more, just until the greens are wilted.

Dandelion

Dandelion, of course, is an age-old spring tonic. I was first instructed in its rejuvenating powers when I lived down south. Miss Glover was a picture of contentment, though by the standards of most of the world she had little to crow about. She never had much more than a little cottage to her name, but it was neatly and proudly decorated with wonderful gewgaws and antiques handed down from the time her grandmother was a slave, or as castoffs from her various employers when she worked as a maid. I would try to visit with her at least once a week, falling into one of her red velvet chairs that stood sentry beside a large black stove in her front room ("That's called a lady's chair," she drawled as I slumped into one of them, wearing torn jeans and an old T-shirt. "'Cause your skirt spreads out so pretty on either side of you."). Most of what she told me—a quiet girl of twenty—left me breathless with wonder at the sheer volume of audacious willpower that got her small body through a lifetime of trial and tribulation.

One day near the end of March, she invited me over for lunch. I knocked on her door, but received no response. She had asked me over for lunch so I knew she was expecting me. I was contemplating cutting through her window screen for fear she may have collapsed or even be dead inside. But before I could act, she came slowly waltzing up the steps, carrying a bag in one hand and sprigs of a woody plant with white blossoms in the other. I greeted her with relief and took the bag, asking her where she'd been.

"It's cotton blossom time," she announced, as I followed her into the kitchen, where her shopping bag had spilled out its contents of green leaves and yellow flowers.

"That's our lunch. Gonna fix us up for spring," Miss Glover said with real relish as she arranged the cotton branches in a vase then carried it into the living room, where she put it on top of the cold black stove between the two lady's chairs.

I looked at the greens—the exact same ones I was forced to pull from the garden when I was young. I knew them as piss-weeds and didn't see how in the name of God I was going to eat them, but you just didn't say no to Miss Glover. I stood beside her at the sink as she sorted through the leaves, choosing only the smallest and rinsing them under the faucet while placing the bigger leaves to the side. She washed the small leaves again, then patted them dry. Next, she took out a big black cast-iron frying pan and lightly sautéed some fresh bacon (and I mean fresh-cured, from a pig she knew personally), then threw in the greens, turning them twice to wilt and spooning them out into two bowls with a slotted spoon. A few bacon crisps came with the greens, which she then sprinkled with cider vinegar, a little salt, and a few twists from the peppermill. Miss Glover carried the bowls to the table, set out glasses of fresh iced tea, then motioned for me to sit across from her. After a short prayer, she dug into the salad and I followed suit, surprisingly happy with the dish—smoothly bitter, slightly astringent. I immediately felt somehow lighter.

"Good for the kidneys, passes all that poison through your water," Miss Glover commented bluntly. For one solid week in March (timing for picking dandelions depends on whether it's an early or late spring, or, for Miss Glover, when the cotton blossomed in the fields), Miss Glover consumed nothing but dandelions—salads, soups, teas. She ate not just the leaves but the flower heads (shredded) and the roots (scrubbed clean and chewed slowly like gum). With the dandelions she drank water, sometimes very sweet iced tea (made from red clover, sassafras, or ground ivy), which she claimed further detoxified the blood and strengthened the kidneys.

You don't argue with a woman who's reached her ninth decade without a serious ailment. From that time on, whenever spring rolls around I've tried to follow her directions. Since I live up north, I don't have access to a cotton field to gauge when the time is right, but I generally start eating what my family calls my dandelion messes—usually a course of salads—around the week of May 10.

DANDELION SALAD

Makes 2 servings

1 bunch fresh young dandelion leaves, coarsely shredded

4 strips bacon or prosciutto

1 firm Vidalia onion, cut into thin slices (see Note)

Salt and pepper

3 to 4 tablespoons good cider vinegar or herb-flavored vinegar

Sort through the dandelion leaves and discard stems and any leaves that seem tough. Wash well, dry, and place them in a large salad bowl.

Sauté the bacon or prosciutto in a skillet until crisp. Add the onion slices and cook briefly, turning once or twice just to wilt. Remove the bacon and onions with a slotted spoon and mix with the dandelion leaves, tossing briefly. (You don't want to drain the bacon and onions, but let the grease gently coat—not drown—the leaves.)

Sprinkle the salad with salt and pepper to taste and the vinegar.

Note: As I have mention earlier, onions themselves, are considered a potent cleanser and I've heard testimony from people whom I consider to be quite sane who say they get a shipment of Vidalia onions every spring (they're available usually from March to June) and eat them—raw—to strengthen their blood and improve their circulation. Vidalia onions have a sweet, juicy flavor so you can get away with this without burning your mouth and guts. If you can't find Vidalias for the salad, leeks and Bermuda or red onions are good substitutes.

. . .

Miss Glover made dandelion wine from the reserved bigger leaves. She bottled the wine in good quantity and used it through the winter whenever she felt herself growing sluggish. She added a table-spoon or two to cups of tea when her arthritis acted up, and sipped a small cordial glass of wine before she went to bed (on the theory that it helped her body work through the night while she slept); she gave me a glass a couple of times when she knew I was suffering from menstrual cramps (and it did, indeed, seem to help).

I've been trying to find a recipe that duplicates the taste of Miss Glover's pale green white, slightly rough, earthy-tasting wine, which also had a smooth little kick to it. The nearest I've found is this one, adapted from *Directions for Cookery* by Miss Eliza Leslie (1828).

DANDELION WINE

Fills four 750-ml wine bottles

4 cups dandelion leaves and flowers

3 pounds sugar (about 7½ cups)

1 tablespoon granulated yeast

3 beaten egg whites, optional

2 pounds raisins (about 6 cups), optional

Wash the dandelion leaves and flowers under a stream of cold water to remove any dirt. Very gently shred the leaves and flowers (be careful not to lose too much juice as you cut through the leaves). Set aside in a large earthenware bowl or jug (see Note).

Bring 1 gallon pure spring water and the sugar to a boil in a large soup pot, stirring until the sugar is thoroughly dissolved. Pour the sugar water over the dandelions and let stand until cool. Mix in the yeast and stir until the yeast is thoroughly dissolved. Cover the container with a heavy tea towel and let ferment for 3 days in a cool place.

After 3 days, strain the liquid through a fine sieve. You can further clarify the wine by mixing in the beaten egg whites, then scooping them out (the egg whites act like a sponge that attracts any remaining scum particles). Pour the strained and clarified liquid into a large earthenware jug or bowl with a tight-fitting lid. Add raisins if you want a stronger fermentation to take place (raisins also sweeten the wine). Cover tightly and let rest for 6 months. The wine is now ready to be bottled and served.

Note: Avoid plastic or metal bowls which impart a metallic taste to the wine.

⋙ SULPHUR AND TREACLE ⋘

(This recipe is included for its historical relevance only.
*It is **not** recommended for modern-day use.)*

Makes 1 cup

A rather stern-sounding tonic is recommended in *The Scottish Bakehouse Cook Book.* It has the Cotton Mather title of "Sulphur and Treacle." The sulfur called for in this recipe refers to brimstone, and it is horrible—foul tasting and hard on the digestive tract. Treacle is a molasseslike substance; it is a syrupy by-product of sugar refining. If you're willing to give this a try and can't find treacle (I'm told it's available in England), use Golden Syrup (a light molasses) instead.

2 tablespoons sulphur	Mix these together and take a spoonful once a day. (It is also reported to be good for clearing the face of spots and pimples when rubbed into the skin.)
1 cup treacle	

. . .

SULFUR WAS BELIEVED to burn impurities from the blood. A better ingredient for that, I think, is the vinegar used in the next two tonics. They are similar preparations but were believed to do two very
different things. The first is an old Amish tonic, used not only in the
spring but also any time a little weight loss is desired (not an unusual
request after heavy winter food).

GENERAL TONIC

Makes 1 serving

1 tablespoon fresh
cider vinegar

1 teaspoon honey

Mix the vinegar and honey with ½ cup cold
water in a tall glass. Drink in the morning.
This is recommended not only as an appetite
suppressant but for kidney troubles and
hay fever.

. . .

DR. ROBERT WALLACE JOHNSON recommended this drink to add oxygen to the blood—a theory that probably does not stand up to scientific proof.

OXYCRATE

Makes 1 generous quart

¼ cup white wine vinegar

1½ tablespoons honey

Mix the vinegar and honey with 4 cups of water in a bottle and cork.

Take 1 tablespoon in the morning.

May also be used to rub on sore joints (!).

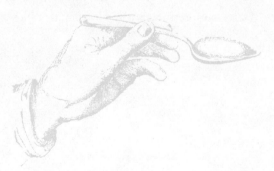

❧ ROBIN RESTORATIVE ❧

*(This recipe is included for its historical relevance only.
It is **not** recommended for modern-day use.)*

Makes 1 serving

Winter tonics are usually a little more filling. They add bulk
to replenish any weight loss or wear and tear on the body after the summer's hard agricultural work.

A quite charming winter tonic is from Mary Boland Pequignot's *A Handbook of Invalid Cooking* (1893). She recommended
a course of eating robins before they fly south. My secret belief is that she thought of these harbingers of spring as rich
in vitality and, by eating them through the autumn months,
the human body would absorb some of their freshness.

2 robins, plucked and dressed	Preheat the oven to 475°F.
Salt and pepper	Wash the robins and pat dry. Sprinkle with a little salt and pepper, then wrap each in a slice of bacon. Place in a roasting pan and roast for 8 to 10 minutes.
2 slices fresh bacon	Increase heat to broil and place the robins under the broiler for 4 more minutes, or until the skin and bacon are crisp.

. . .

SHELLFISH WERE ALSO CONSIDERED a good winter preparation. Shrimp, especially, were prized—so much so that Dr. Robert Wallace Johnson recommended carrying a package of sautéed shrimp around in your pocket and nibbling them through the month of September. His one stipulation was that the shells be eaten, as well. The recommended course is to consume a serving once a day to commence as soon as the air chills and sweetens.

A COURSE FOR WINTER

Makes 1 serving

About 1 cup fresh shrimp, shells and heads attached

2 tablespoons coarsely ground black pepper

2 tablespoons best-quality olive oil

Wash the shrimp well and pat dry. Press the pepper into the shrimp with the palm of your hand, trying to get as much pepper as possible to stick to the shells.

Heat the olive oil in a large skillet. Add the shrimp and cook quickly, stirring until the shells turn bright pink. Remove at once to a plate. Before serving, the heads may be removed. Eat hot or cold.

. . .

ANOTHER SHELLFISH TONIC was recorded by Brillat-Savarin, by way of M. F. K. Fisher in *A Cordiall Water.* He called it "A Restorative" for "people of unstable and vacillating temperament." I tried it out during a week when my endearingly wayward teenage son was doing his best to make my husband and me feel unstable. It took me a full day to prepare the dish—from shopping for the ingredients to the final straining—and by the time it was ready, I was pretty wiped out. Brillat-Savarin carefully admonishes the reader to drink the restorative only in the morning, 2 hours before breakfast, so that's what we did for the next few days. While Sam continues to be a healthy teenager, his parents, I'm happy to report, are feeling a little more on solid ground.

BRILLAT-SAVARIN'S RESTORATIVE

Makes about 1 week's supply for 2 people

12 tablespoons (1½ sticks) sweet butter

1 veal knuckle (about 2 pounds), cut in quarters lengthwise

4 medium onions, quartered

1 cup watercress leaves

Melt ⅔ stick of the butter in a large soup pot. Add the veal knuckle, onions, and watercress and cook, stirring, until the knuckle is almost cooked and the onions are nicely browned, about 15 minutes (add more butter if the knuckle is sticking to the pan).

Add 3 quarts water, scraping the bottom of the pot to loosen any meat and onions.

Salt and fresh
pepper

2 Cornish game hens
(see Note)

2 pounds very fresh
crayfish

Bring to a boil, lower to a simmer, and let cook for 2 hours. Remove from the heat and taste the broth. Add salt and pepper to taste. Refrigerate for a few hours or, better yet, overnight. Skim any fat congealed on the top.

Split the hens in half and flatten them with the broad side of a knife. In a large skillet, melt the rest of the butter and brown the hens with the crayfish until the hens are brown and the crayfish are pink. Add the hens and crayfish to the veal stock, scraping the skillet clean. Bring to a rapid boil, then let simmer for 1 hour.

Strain the liquid through a fine sieve and then again through cheesecloth. Let cool. You can serve the hens and crayfish as a meal, but the restorative is just the broth. Take about 4 ounces of the broth 2 hours before breakfast in the morning. (The hens and crayfish are particularly delicious over buttered noodles or good rice.)

Note: I've faithfully interpreted Brillat-Savarin's recipe except for the fact that it calls for old pigeons instead of game hens. If you can find pigeons or squabs—young or old—substitute them.

· · ·

TWO YEAR-ROUND TONICS—one strictly for morning and the other to be taken both morning and night—are little vitamin-packed sips. Their effectiveness depends upon how they are administered—both must be taken while still in bed, the small quantity sipped slowly. The body must then remain still for at least 10 minutes. If nothing else, these tonics offer a pleasant way to start and end the day, reason enough to benefit from them.

A YEAR-ROUND TONIC

Makes about six ½-cup servings

1 cup fresh sage blossoms (usually blooms in late July)

Peel from 1 lemon

3 cups good-quality bourbon

Collect and dry the sage blossoms as they appear. When you have enough, pack them and the lemon peel in a glass jar and pour on the bourbon. Cover tightly and let stand at least 2 weeks (the longer the better).

Take 1 small cordial glass first thing in the morning (rest for 15 minutes with eyes closed before standing) and last thing at night.

. . .

THIS RECIPE comes from a friend's grandmother who took it without any sweeteners up until the morning she died at the age of 93. As good a testament as that is, I would nevertheless add a tablespoon or two of honey, simply because I don't like to pucker my insides that early in the day. In *A Cordiall Water* M. F. K. Fisher mentions a similar drink using grapefruit instead of lemons. Pink grapefruits prepared this way are, indeed, a bracing way to start the morning and probably don't need the addition of sweeteners.

A MORNING TONIC

Makes 1 serving

1 lemon

At night, chop the lemon, skin and all, into small chunks. Place in a bowl and cover with 1 cup boiling water. Let sit overnight.

In the morning, strain off the liquid into a glass. Dispose of the fruit pulp and drink.

The Black Suit

Two Christmases ago, my mother-in-law, Sally, told my husband she wanted to buy me something expensive.

"Something to wear," she specified. When Chris asked her why, she simply stated that it would make her happy. Tales about Sally inevitably began with what she was wearing; thin and shapely, she was a firm believer in the transforming power of glamour.

"I'm not suppose to tell you this, but she hates how you dress," Chris laughed when he informed me of her wishes. I'd known this for a long time—a woman who loved Bergdorf Goodman's, she could never quite fathom my reliance on the Salvation Army. But she was kind and open-minded and only on a few occasions did she let out that my clothes offended her sensibilities. In truth, her response to my wardrobe became an unspoken amusement for me and a silent, tactfully-born burden for her.

Now, she decided, she was going to do something about it.

"Have you gone shopping yet?" She asked me a few weeks later.

"Not yet," I admitted rather sheepishly.

"Well, tell me what you want and I'll look."

"I don't know. I don't really need anything."

"Think," she commanded sharply.

"Okay, a jacket, a black jacket."

"Fine," she capitulated. "I'll start looking tomorrow."

But she never did. She had recovered from surgery for breast cancer ten years before and carried on with her life, working, traveling, gardening, and giving splendid parties with very tough-minded women she called her "fellow crones." But then spots appeared on her x-rays; exploratory surgery confirmed that one lung and a few lymph nodes would have to go. Through the late winter and early spring that year, her body grew weaker. Her doctors thought the cancer might have spread into her bones, but they weren't sure. Treatments became more aggressive. Yet, she insisted on continuing as if nothing was wrong. She made plans for us to visit her and attend a large family dinner over the Easter holiday. Sally willed herself into a white linen pants suit and made up her face so that her white skin glowed with a semblance of health. She got through the day, collapsed in exhaustion the next, and complained to me right before we were leaving that we hadn't gone shopping.

"Now, you'll just have to do this for me," she said firmly after I kissed her goodbye.

I didn't, though, too busy with work, with the things I was writing, with my children and husband, and with my own parents who were ailing. Shopping for a present for myself was far down the list of my daily chores.

And that was how things stood until the summer. Sally was getting weaker; Chris' brother, Tim, who lived near her and oversaw her care, was tired. Since Chris couldn't manage an extended time away from his job until late in the fall, we decided that, with my more flexible work schedule, I would go out and help Sally for a week.

"Perfect," she replied when we told her I was coming. "We'll go shopping."

When she met me at the airport, I couldn't believe she had made it that far—she was like a blossom-heavy flower, her thin body tethered to the support of an ornately carved rosewood cane. The drive to her house was interminable and scary, the high doses of morphine she took making her judgment on the highway less than sound.

Once we were finally home and she was lying comfortably on her couch while I searched the liquor cabinet for a stiff drink, Sally announced, "We'll go to Saks first thing tomorrow."

Shocked by Sally's frailty, I thought it was foolish to even consider such an outing, but she was strong-willed. I cooked a special dinner that night. I boiled new potatoes in milk to ease the pain in her stomach, sauteed calves liver in wine to give her strength, steamed plums for dessert to alleviate her constipation. Finally, I brewed her a hot toddy of weak camomile tea, two tablespoons of milk, and a good-size dollop of honey. I changed the sheets on her bed, plumped up her pillows, then helped Sally into bed and kissed her good night.

She slept through to 8 the next morning, reporting that it had been months since she had such a good night's sleep. It's the food, I thought, feeling so satisfied with myself while I cooked her a pot of oatmeal for breakfast. I was sure I could get her feeling better again and she, too, seemed to take heart that something as simple as a course of good food would set her on the road to health again. We got dressed in a celebratory mood, then headed out.

Soon after walking inside the vast mall, Sally began to look for a bench to sit down. Her legs were giving out and she wanted to take something for the pain in her hip. She took two aspirins, drank a little water, then we started off again, only to crumple at the next bench where she took another aspirin and drank a little more water. When we finally got to the store, she collapsed into the pillows of a deep love seat.

She waved off my concern. "Start looking," she commanded and I obeyed, trailing through racks of designer labels until I found the perfect black jacket.

"And what goes with it?" She turned to ask the saleswoman who quickly scurried off to gather up several different skirts and pants of varying style. The jacket was already close to $800 and I did the math for everything else. With either skirt or pants, I would have $1,500 worth of clothes on, not including shirt and shoes—more than I ever wore before. Sally handed the saleswoman her credit card.

"We're taking the jacket, the long skirt, the narrow pants, and two of the re-embroidered lace blouses over there, one small and the other medium," she said, then turned to me. "We'll go out to tea tomorrow at the Ritz and show off our new things."

She was happy, actually thrilled, as I struggled with the garment bags while supporting her back through the mall to the car. She let me drive her home and, after taking a few spoonfuls of a custard I had made, she laid down for a nap. A few hours later she woke up in such pain that I gave her an extra dose of morphine that knocked her out until midnight.

We never made it out to tea, nor to any of the other events she planned that week. The next day, with her stomach still unsettled, I steeped a pot of ginger tea and made a clear veal consommé. Then she sent me off to the video store to rent a movie. Thinking we could both use something frivolous, I picked up *The Women*. Sally was delighted with the choice, but it took us three days and nights to finish. Sometimes, she was in so much pain she closed her eyes and wanted only silence. I would hold her hands, cover her in the mohair throw she kept by the couch. When we did watch the movie, we talked about the costumes, those rich concoctions of feminine perfection the actresses wore, all frills and trains and corsets and feathered hats that got them through their man-troubles in splendid style. Sally had worn things like that and lamented that she had given them away or worn them to shreds.

"I sure was something," she smiled, cocking her head at a proud angle while describing a short lamb-skin jacket she once paired with a long lace skirt.

Meantime, when I wasn't looking after Sally, I was cooking her things—every dish I knew, every elixir I could remember; but nothing really worked.

"Delicious," she would whisper and I'd carry the hardly touched dish back into the kitchen with tears in my eyes.

SALLY DIED in my husband's arms the following March. At the memorial service, I sat in the front row wearing the beautiful black suit she bought for me. While my husband, his father, and Sally's friends talked about her life, I thought of our week together, wishing I could have brought her more comfort, relieved the pain, erased all her anxiety. With my little goblets of wine jelly and small chicken cro-quettes surrounded by tiny peaks of garlic mashed potatoes, I should have been able to shield her better from death's stare but I had failed, and I was angry.

And yet, as time has melted my sorrow to merely an ache, I've come to realize that the dishes I prepared for her did all that they were meant to do. In another time, when people were more mindful of their mortality, invalid food was simply meant to bring a small drop of consolation—both to the family and the dying. While I cooked for Sally, I did feel I was doing something useful for her and, while she ate, she felt less removed from the world. Her weak body received nourishment and my sore heart was eased. Over bowls of soup and fresh teas, we laughed and gossiped, whispered secrets and feelings we would not have otherwise shared. Our love and understanding of each other intensified and, at the end of the day, this was all I could have hoped for.

I still do not wear the suit very often. But when I do, I know that I look as perfect as I'll ever be and that assurance braces me to face the world with just a little more certainty and grace. Sometimes, when I am rummaging for something to wear, I spy its richness among my plainer clothes and smile, hearing Sally softly chiding me as I was leaving her with the suit wrapped safely in its garment bag.

"Comfort comes in many forms, dear," she said.

I do believe I know that now.

Bibliography

A full bibliography of invalid cooking would take many pages. There is, however, an essential core group of recipes that make up the most important part of feeding the sick. These are the books I have used as source material.

BIOGRAPHY:

Strachey, Lytton. *Eminent Victorians.* 1918. Reprint. New York: Harvest/Harcourt Brace Jovanovich, Publishers.

Woodham-Smith, Cecil. *Florence Nightingale, 1820–1910.* New York: McGraw Hill Book Company, Inc. 1951.

HISTORICAL BACKGROUND:

Beck, Amanda K. *Reference Hand Book for Nurses.* Philadelphia: W. B. Sounders Co. 1905.

Beecher, Catharine Esther. *The American Woman's Home.* 1869. Reprint. Hartford, CT.: Stowe-Day Foundation. 1975.

Beeton, Mrs. *The Book of Household Management.* Reprint. New York: Farrar, Strauss & Giroux, Inc. 1969.

Byler, Emma. *Plain & Happy Living.* Cleveland: Goosefoot Acres Press. 1991.

Humphreys, Frederick, Dr. *Humphreys' Mentor and Medical Advisor.* New York: Humphreys' Homeopathy Medicine Co. 1891.

Jamison, Alcinous B., Dr. *Intestinal Ills.* New York: Charles A. Tyrrell. 1901.

Markham, Gervase. *The English Housewife.* 1615. Reprint. Kingston, Ontario, Canada: McGill University Press. 1986.

Newcomer, Marian, Dr. *Bewildered Patient.* Boston: Hale, Cushman & Flint. 1936.

Nightingale, Florence. *Notes on Nursing: What It Is and What It Is Not.* 1860. Reprint. New York: Dover Publications, Inc. 1969.

Price Herndle, Diane. *Invalid Women; Figuring Feminine Illness in American Fiction and Culture, 1840–1940.* Chapel Hill, N.C.: University of North Caroline Press, Chapel Hill, 1983.

Soyer, Alexis. *A Culinary Campaign.* 1857. Reprint. Lewes, England: Southover. 1995.

Soyer, Alexis. *Memoirs of Alexis Soyer.* 1859. Reprint. Rottingdean, Sussex, England: Cooks Books. 1985.

Weil, Andrew. *Spontaneous Healing.* New York: Alfred A. Knopf, Inc. 1995.

COOKBOOKS:

Bradley, Martha. *The British Housewife or the Cook, Housekeeper, and Gardiner's Companion.* London: S. Crowder and H. Woodgate. 1770.

Chase, A. W., Dr. *Information for Everybody: An Invaluable Collection of About 800 Practical Recipes.* Ann Arbor: Self-published. 1866.

Farmer, Fannie Merritt. *Food and Cookery for the Sick and Convalescent.* Boston: Little, Brown and Co. 1904.

Fisher, M. F. K. *A Cordiall Water.* Boston: Little, Brown and Co. 1961.

Fothergill, John Milner, Dr. *Food for the Invalid; The Convalescent; The Dyspeptic; and The Gouty.* New York: Macmillan and Co. 1880.

Grieve, Mrs. M. *A Modern Herbal.* 1931. Reprint. New York: Dover Publications, Inc. 1971.

Hall, William W., Dr. *Health by Good Living*. New York: Hurd and Houghton. 1870.

Harland, Marion (AKA Mary Virginia Hawes Terhune). *The New Common Sense in the Household*. New York: Frederick A. Stokes Co. 1926.

Henderson, Mary Newton Foote. *Diet for the Sick*. New York: Harper & Brothers. 1885.

Howard, Maria Willett. *Lowney's Cook Book*. Boston: Walter M. Lowney Co. 1912.

Johnson, Robert Wallace, Dr. *The Nurse's Guide and Family Assistant*. Philadelphia: Anthony Finley. 1819.

Kellar, Jane Carpenter, Ellen Miller, and Paul Stambach, ed. *Selected Receipts of a Van Rensselaer Family 1785–1835*. Albany, N.Y.: Historic Cherry Hill. 1976.

Leslie, Eliza. *Directions for Cookery in Its Various Branches*. 1828. Reprint. New York: Arno Press. 1973.

Little, May. *A Year's Dinners*. London: Harrod's LTD. 1930.

Pequignot, Mary A. Boland. *A Handbook of Invalid Cooking*. New York: The Century Co. 1893.

Pitkin, Eliza A. *Invalid Cookery*. Chicago: E. A. Pitkin. 1880.

Sachse, Helena V. *How to Cook for the Sick*. Philadelphia: Lippincott. 1901.

Soyer, Alexis. *The Modern Housewife*. New York: D. Appleton. 1859.

Soyer, Alexis. *Soyer's Cookery Book*. 1854. Reprint. New York: D. McKay Co. 1959.

Tantaquidgeon, Gladys. *Folk Medicine of the Delaware and Related Algonkian Indians*. Harrisburg: Pennsylvania Historical and Museum Commission. 1972.

Terhune, Mary Virginia Hawes. *Common Sense in the Household*. New York: C. Scribner & Co., Inc. 1871.

Thompson, Margaret J. *Food for the Sick and Well*. Yonkers-on-Hudson, N.Y.: World Book Co. 1920.

Wallace, Lily Haxworth. *The Rumford Complete Cook Book*. Providence, R.I.: The Rumford Co. 1908.

White, Isabella M. *The Scottish Bakehouse Cook Book*, 3rd edition. Martha's Vineyard, MA.: The Tashmoo Press. 1979.

Index